Praise for *The Yoga Manifesto*:

'An important read for anyone who rolls out their mat.'

Stylist

'A confessional memoir and meticulous polemic.'

Kate Spicer, journalist *The Sunday Times*

'*The Yoga Manifesto* is about equality, creativity and revolu-
tionary hope – and you definitely don't need to practise yoga
to know these things matter.'

Stella Duffy, author of *Lullaby Beach*

'The first yoga book I've read with a punk rock attitude. Nadia
is a formidable storyteller taking us through the highs and
lows of her personal journey. However most critical is her
fierce analysis of the appropriation of yoga.'

Sima Kumar, co-founder of The Other Box

'A brilliantly honest account of navigating the yoga industry
and its highs and lows. A must read.'

Lorna Fisher, yoga teacher @dynamicflowyoga

NADIA GILANI

THE
YOGA
MANIFESTO

How Yoga Helped Me and
Why It Needs to Save Itself

bluebird
books for life

First published 2022 by Bluebird

This paperback edition first published 2023 by Bluebird
an imprint of Pan Macmillan
The Smithson, 6 Briset Street, London EC1M 5NR
EU representative: Macmillan Publishers Ireland Ltd, 1st Floor,
The Liffey Trust Centre, 117–126 Sheriff Street Upper,
Dublin 1, D01 YC43
Associated companies throughout the world
www.panmacmillan.com

ISBN 978-1-5290-6514-5

Pan Macmillan does not have any control over, or any responsibility for,
any author or third-party websites referred to in or on this book.

1 3 5 7 9 8 6 4 2

A CIP catalogue record for this book is available from the British Library.

Typeset by Palimpsest Book Production Ltd, Falkirk, Stirlingshire
Printed and bound by CPI Group (UK) Ltd, Croydon, CR0 4YY

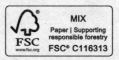

Visit **www.panmacmillan.com/bluebird** to read more about all our books
and to buy them. You will also find features, author interviews and
news of any author events, and you can sign up for e-newsletters
so that you're always first to hear about our new releases.

CONTENT WARNING

This book includes experiences of eating disorders, alcohol dependency, domestic violence, suicidal thoughts and sexual violence that some readers might find upsetting.

For Jameela Khatoon Ali and Tasneem Gilani

Contents

Introduction:
Viv Made Me Do It

Viv Albertine, guitarist for 1970s British punk band The Slits told me how to write this book. Kind of. I met her on a creative writing course run by the Arvon Foundation in 2015. The course ran over five days and on the third day, a guest author was invited to join us and share their work. Viv was there for that.

I had ended up on the course because I needed a break. I had decided to look upon it as a retreat and form of healing because after many years of troubles with food and alcohol and almost a decade of working as a news journalist, I was exhausted. I needed a rest but was also searching for some serious discipline in what had otherwise been a chaotic life for too long.

I didn't quite arrive prepared. Everyone else seemed to have come with a burning idea of what they wanted to write about – except me. But I wasn't worried. I had enough experience of living by the seat of my pants and assumed that some of Viv's genius might inspire and send me on my way. To a certain extent I wasn't wrong. On the course, we were put in groups that each took it in turn to cook dinner on different days. I was red-faced stirring a vegan risotto in the kitchen one evening when I spotted Viv wearing skinny jeans, a cropped jacket and spiky-heeled boots, leaning against the dining room doorway. I was immediately starstruck and then felt crushed. I knew I wouldn't be brave enough to talk to her as I had hoped. I shuffled to one end of the dining table and stared at the salad on my plate, hoping she wouldn't notice me. But she sat next to me, didn't she? And that's when everything changed.

Viv asked what I was writing. 'Lots,' I said. 'How do I turn it into a book?' I asked. 'Do what I do,' she told me. 'Write it all in short bits and move it around later.' It took a while for me to understand what Viv meant, and I didn't actually write anything for several years, but when I started this book I remembered her advice. The chapters in Viv's first book *Clothes, Music, Boys* are exceptionally short. This method had clearly worked for her. So I did the same – wrote a bunch of stories and threaded them together later. A bit like taking a set of yoga poses and linking them with a series of flowing movements (more on that soon). This is what you've got in your hands now.

What you're holding isn't an expert's how-to-do-yoga book, nor is it a tips-and-tricks guide to building a yoga career. I'm not qualified to do either of those things. I'm just someone who has practised yoga in some shape or form for a long time. This book is about that and some of the crazy things that happened along the way. It's also about the wonderful, strange, awkward and sometimes downright weird things I have learnt from working as a yoga teacher. I have a long history with yoga in my life and it hasn't always been an easy ride. I'm here to tell you what yoga has meant to me, and how I've seen it help others. In particular, those I've had the privilege to teach who are so often ignored by the wellness industry that yoga has got itself wrapped up in. It's about struggling to exist in a paradox: living and working in what's become a self-care industry, which left me feeling uncared for at many times.

But there's hope, because this book is also about the ways I learnt even more about what yoga could mean for me by helping others apply it to their own lives. I hope I can help you in some way with this book too. I care deeply about doing this because yoga has a special place in my heart. I was introduced to the practice early in life and I'd like to help more people find it too. It might seem like that job's already been done because yoga appears to be everywhere and everyone seems to be doing it. Even if you've never set foot in a class, I'm guessing that you've seen someone hugging a mat on their way to one.

On social media it's hard to get past a few scrolls without being bombarded with advertisements for the latest activewear, props and equipment, or for workshops on how to build a yoga business. If you haven't got a clue what I'm talking about – keep looking, it won't take long. Like magic mushrooms in a field in September, once you see one, you begin to see millions. This yoga boom is a zeitgeist I didn't see coming when I first got on a shabby mat in an old community gym in 1996 when this practice was still obscure, seen as alternative, somewhat radical even. Thankfully there are still grassroots yoga projects and events like that going on locally outside big cities, which means plenty of people are still able to enjoy a yoga practice in village halls, leisure centres, and other community spaces. It's true too that many of these people are deeply engaged in yoga beyond merely the physical aspects of the practice (there's way more to it, which I'll get to) and are not in thrall to big business. It's just a shame that this isn't the zeitgeist. Don't get me wrong, for yoga to be available to the masses is a good thing. There's clearly a huge need for it as an antidote to our frenetic modern-day lives. But at times it feels like it's coming at a cost.

I've practised yoga for more than twenty-five years. It's a practice I have a profound relationship with, but this has come after many years of getting it wrong. Yoga has somehow seen me through various scrapes in life: from attending classes drunker than I thought I was, head standing in toilets in office jobs to cure hangovers and chain-smoking roll-ups while training to be a yoga teacher. So the practice has never been a miracle cure when the chips were down for me and there were certainly times I wanted to give up on yoga but perhaps it didn't want to give up on me. We're still together today but it's safe to say that yoga and I had a complicated relationship for a long time.

Yoga is most famous for its postures but there is so much more to it than that. The poses make those of us who practise feel good and they facilitate an emotional and spiritual shift if we're lucky, but there is a deeper meaning to all of that too. I didn't know it when I first discovered yoga as a teenager, but this ancient scientific, psychological and philosophical system was originally intended as a method for self-inquiry and a way to experience oneness with a universal conscious-ness. The postures prepare our bodies to meditate and as we do that, we learn about ourselves. For me the practice is also about learning how to live with joy and ease, both things that haven't come easy to me and in this book I'll tell you why. Meditation might feel impossible – scary even – particularly for anxious, depressed, and restless people or those who have leaned on various unhelpful crutches like I have. I found it practically impossible to sit still at first, but that was okay.

The aim is only ever to practise and see what we find. When I think about yoga like that it opens up endless possibilities that are far more compelling than being able to do a handstand (though of course practising that is fun too).

Most importantly, yoga works – as a tool to benefit our bodies and minds – when we believe that it will work. As we practise, we discover who we are, what's in our heart of hearts and what's worth living for. That's what I've found it to do for me over the years. There's more, but that's the crux. Since I haven't always found yoga or indeed life to be straightforward, I'm interested in exploring how we all find our way through both. It's going to be different for everyone but what I've discovered is that most of us need something to believe in. Religion might be one path, career another. Relationships tend to help, and addictions and destructive behaviours (which I know a fair bit about) can keep us going for a while too. Then there's yoga, which has been many things for me at the same time: a faith, discipline, friend, and an all-encompassing lifestyle, but also something I've been at odds with at times before falling in love with it all over again.

My relationship with yoga became even more confusing when I found myself working inside the yoga business as a teacher. I wasn't quite expecting yoga teaching to throw up big questions about my identity, the world and life itself. The biggest issue I faced was that the wellness industry I was working within seemed to contradict the practice I had known all my life. The industry looked increasingly to me like a giant myth that had less to do with real yoga as I understood it than it claimed it did. I found myself wanting to get back to the truth. This is why I wrote this book: to explore the deeper questions about where yoga has come from, what it now means to me and other practitioners given all I've been through and where it appears to be heading next. I'll present yoga as a political issue and show how for it to be authentic but also stay relevant it must be practised in a way that is engaged in issues facing the world. Looking at yoga in the context of modern life in this way isn't to demolish the past but to ensure it keeps evolving as it always has as well as making sure that it's easy to access for as many people as possible. I'll also be taking aim at the billion-dollar wellness industry to reveal what lies beneath the airbrushed aesthetic of slim-limbed bendy practitioners sporting bum-sculpting leggings that dominates yoga's image worldwide.

A big question I had when I was a new yoga teacher was: how did an ancient practice come to this? I'll be seeking to answer this by exploring how yoga has gone mainstream (which is great), but the fact that it has been white-washed, distorted by Western imperialists and repackaged in platitudinal 'love and light' slogans is a big problem for everyone. I'm not suggesting that yoga should be practised exactly as it was thousands of years ago – far from it. I'd say that my own approach to yoga is fairly liberal because I've had a complex life. Adapting the practice is how I've had to make it work for me, much in the same way anyone who follows a religion will practise it in a way that makes sense to them. But my own contemporary approach doesn't mean I ignore the roots of the practice or the fundamental principles behind what it was designed for. It's this process of reflecting on the past and analyzing the current state of play within yoga that uncovered what seemed to me to be a necessary manifesto for the future. I will be critical in this book at times, but I'll also be showing you that it's not all bad news for yoga, as my own personal relationship and fierce love for this spiritual practice is what's really at the heart of this story I'm about to tell. It's this passion for the practice that gives me hope for what's to come.

I've tried to write a book that no one else has, a book that would have been handy to have when I first started teaching yoga. But this book isn't only for teachers or those working within the yoga industry, it's also for yoga practitioners (or students really), especially beginners – so if that's you, welcome, you're in the right place. This is why I'll be balancing an examination of what I've seen happen to yoga over the years by sharing my changing experiences of the practice with you as I've never seen my own story reflected anywhere else.

By the way, I'm not here to tell you how to practise yoga because there's no single way to do it and I'd be suspicious of anyone who tells you otherwise. This practice can be wonderful and it should be available for you – and I – to make our own however we choose. That's the only way to have a profound and meaningful practice in the end. But I want you to see an honest picture of yoga, what it's become and how it relates to modern life – that's what interests me most, because doing that is what gives the practice a purpose and makes it even better. I'd also like you – especially if you've absent-mindedly picked up this book thinking yoga isn't for you (because of the often-unhelpful ways yoga is marketed) – to stay with me on this journey because I didn't think it was for me when I first started either. But the truth is there's no reason why it can't work for you or anyone.

When Viv Albertine signed my copy of her book, she wrote: *To Nadia, from Viv. Write! Write! Write!* So that's what I've done. I hope you enjoy it, whether you're a long-standing yoga student, interested in getting started or just curious about what the practice can mean for us all on a personal level, but also what it might mean for the modern world we all live in.

CHAPTER 1

Lost in Yoga

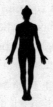

It was November, a week before my birthday and I was heading to work as everyone else went home. *Why had I agreed to do this?* I couldn't remember. I have a history of taking wrong turns in life that have ended in disaster around my birthday and was starting to wonder if this might be the latest one. Gil Scott-Heron's 'Lady Day and John Coltrane' shuffled into my headphones as the train pulled into my stop. 'Ever feel kinda down and out, you don't know just what to do.' *Yeah, I do, Gil*, I thought. 'Livin' all of your days in darkness let the sun shine through'. I walked out of the North London Tube station and caught a glimpse of fireworks far off in the inky black sky. It was a relief to finally be outside. I had just spent an hour fighting my way on and off trains against Monday-night commuters rushing home in the opposite direction. Walking through the underpass at London Bridge Station earlier had felt like being trapped inside a video game. Like dodging bullets, which in this case was everyone else coming at me from all directions.

I was starting to feel anxious about the night ahead, and wondering whether the journey was going to have been worth it. I was on my way to teach a yoga class for refugee boys at a community centre. I had been told that they were aged sixteen to nineteen, so some of them were already young men. I regularly led classes for people from vulnerable communities like this through a charity, but I had not yet taught teenagers. Now that I thought about it, facing a roomful of boys and getting them to do strange things with their bodies was beginning to sound scary. I realized that they might not be interested, just as I hadn't been when I went to my first yoga class. I had been initially drawn to the idea of sharing yoga with these kids because the longer I taught yoga, the more I felt a calling to take the practice to those who might not otherwise find it. It made me feel useful and gave me a sense of purpose. I wanted to show them some resources to help them, like yoga had worked for me. If they weren't interested, then never mind. It was worth a try. Teenagers could be cruel though, couldn't they? I wasn't exactly great company when I was their age. I hadn't thought this through.

The nagging feeling in my gut was telling the truth, because I was about to embark on one of the hardest classes I'd taught up to that point. I had agreed to take this class several months earlier and thought at the time that – cultural, language barriers and life circumstances aside – these boys and I might actually have some things in common. Unlike me, they were in a country they couldn't call home with a government that had a track record for hostile policies against immigrants. I knew that I had been afforded every imaginable privilege that they were not. But there were parallels. Like them, I hadn't had the simplest home life growing up and I was a troubled teen when I first stepped on a yoga mat in a creaking YMCA gym way back in 1996. I was taken to that first class by my mum when I was sixteen and had no faith in the future. I had stopped eating like a normal person and it wasn't long before I had started making myself sick. I didn't know anything about eating disorders so didn't know what was wrong with me at the time. My mum had gone to great lengths trying and failing to help me and didn't know what else to do. She thought yoga might work. I was reluctant, but she was persistent. Yoga didn't cure me or give me a better relationship with my body straight away, but somewhere along the line I took to it. Slowly it became a big part of my life and sprinkled some magic into it, even if I didn't immediately understand how. Having yoga in my life also didn't stop me from engaging in other destructive behaviours like binge-drinking as an adult either. But the practice was always there to return to when I felt ready. Maybe I could help these boys find solace in yoga too. Even if only in a small way. I didn't want to go in heavy-handed and try to convert them to anything they weren't interested in, but I could plant a seed like my mum had with me.

Staring at the map on my phone, I turned onto a residential street in a scruffy but elegant neighbourhood. I walked past expensively painted homes with giant shabby-chic bookshelves visible through bay windows. It was so dark and quiet. *Strange place to have a youth club,* I thought. A self-conscious group of teenagers, hoods up, sped past, avoiding eye contact and giving me a wide berth. *Young people are so great,* I thought, *tonight's going to be fun.* I felt a flicker of excitement light up inside me. It didn't last. The knot of angst returned fast. It got bigger and tighter the closer I got to the community centre where I was headed. I tugged my sleeves over cold fingers and rubbed my wet nose.

What if they don't like me? I thought.

What will I do if they laugh at me? I huddled into my scarf.

Oh sod it, here goes, I told myself and walked in.

I found myself in a dark corridor leading to a main hall. I breathed as deeply as I could and pushed open the door. The noise inside was what hit me first: a giant speaker on wheels blasting out hip hop instrumentals that I recognized and liked but the ceiling's way-too-bright lights were glaring down and I wasn't sure about those. There was nowhere to hide. I looked around and saw groups of tall gangly boys showing each other their mobile phone screens, laughing, shouting, pushing and shoving, and youth workers trying to create some order.

Oh God, I hadn't expected so many people. There must be at least twenty kids in here, I thought, and I realized that I knew nothing about any of them. I didn't know which countries they were from – Africa and the Middle East was all I had been told when I had asked the organizers. Such vast geography didn't offer much. I wanted to know more. *How long had they been here? Were they doing okay? Were their families here too? Did they like London? And what were they so enthralled by on their phones?* But they didn't know anything about me either. Who the hell was I, dressed in smart leggings and a posh hoodie, coming in here to tell them what to do? I had no proof that this was what they were thinking but I would have understood if it was.

As I observed the room, I could tell that some of these boisterous kids – wearing tracksuits, low-hanging baggy jeans and large-tongued trainers – saw themselves as rude boys. They reminded me of boys I knew when I was their age. Boys my school friends fancied. Others were quieter, hanging back. A boy named Belal with the kindest face and a firm handshake wrote my name on a label like they all wore to stick on my top. We sat down and he handed me a tangerine from a snack table. I couldn't bring myself to eat it because my stomach was still turning, but I was grateful to him for being there.

Having someone to talk to was helping calm my nerves. Despite my initial sense of feeling overwhelmed, the longer I sat there, smiling in an effort to warm everyone to me, the more I unexpectedly started to feel at home. Teenagers are all the same really: cocky, confident, insecure; asserting their place, but also shying away from it. Some of them were side-eye glancing at me – a foreign face intruding on their space, perhaps trying to work out why I was there. I guessed they might not take to the yoga I had planned after all. But I kept smiling back and hoping I'd find a way.

Two youth workers leading the evening gathered everyone in a circle to kick off proceedings. We played an ice-breaker game that involved crossing our arms and holding hands so that we were entwined. It reminded me of activities we did at Woodcraft Folk clubs I attended as a child. Woodcraft is a bohemian, hippie version of Girls' Brigade and Girl Guides (I went to those too). But Woodcraft Folk was secular, more laidback, and we called adults by their first names like the kids did here. The game was awkward at first but it wasn't long before we were all laughing from tying our arms in knots and becoming friends. I started to relax. *Maybe we could cancel the yoga and do this all night instead. I'd prefer that*, I thought. So I wasn't quite ready when one of the youth leaders announced: 'This is Nadia who is going to do some yoga with us now,' and handed me the floor. Game on.

The jitters came flooding back, my stomach lurched and I felt faint. But there was no time to panic. At least twenty pairs of eyes looked at me expectantly. I asked everyone to collect a mat and it took us ages to get them to line up because some of the boys were acting up or sitting out, stubbornly refusing to help. I flashed back to my own teen years. I had been the same: moody, apprehensive, unpredictable. I had an eye on the clock – we were already 15 minutes behind schedule, so I had to get things going. But with mats in place, half of the boys rushed to the back of the room and sat on the floor against the wall, scrolling through their phones again. Of course, I got it. They didn't know what was going to happen. I represented uncertainty, so getting them to trust me was going to be the first hurdle. A few of them didn't want to take their coats off, others weren't up for removing their shoes. I decided not to push it. I plugged my phone into the speaker, put on some gentle electronic music to assuage any discomfort they might feel with silence and turned around.

'OK, everyone. Let's go,' I said. All I could do was give it a shot.

I felt it best to keep them moving as much as possible, so I taught an hour of Ashtanga Yoga – a dynamic form of doing postures that I have practised for many years. What makes this approach distinct is synching the breath with the movement. With practice the breath starts to initiate the movement and that's when the magic begins to happen. Neuro-scientific research also shows that people who have Post-Traumatic Stress Disorder (PTSD) can benefit from physical practices to help process trauma and improve the resilience of their nervous system. I found out how yoga could specifically help PTSD when I did trauma-awareness training and a tutor from The Minded Institute in London told us evidence showed that breathing and moving in an integrated way could actually shrink the amygdala, the part of the brain that enlarges as a response to trauma. This was one of the reasons I felt so passionate about working with refugees. To show them how to use yoga as a form of self-help and healing.

We were halfway through the first Sun Salutation sequence when the giggles started. I couldn't help but feel myself almost laughing too because, looking at it from their point of view and given that we had only just met, what we were doing was pretty odd. But I remembered my authority, I was the teacher so had to keep myself together. I did my best to cajole them along, walking between their mats and waving my arms to show them the way, exaggerating my movements the way people do when they don't speak your language. 'Breathe out and bend the knee,' I called out, getting them into Warrior Two pose. 'Bend the knee,' I said again when no one responded. 'The knee is bending, more bending, bending more . . .' Everyone's legs were shaking, but I could see that they were strong so I held them there a while longer.

It was helpful that they were all wearing name stickers since I had only briefly spoken to Belal when I arrived. 'Hassan! I think .you can bend it more, no?' I called out, raising my eyebrows and smiling as widely as I could. I knew I was pushing it, but I wanted to see if these teenagers would rise to meet me. Hassan laughed back and I laughed with him. *Good*, I thought, *they know I'm on their side now*. I asked them to inhale and exhale into the same pose on the other side. 'It's your left foot turning outwards, Kwame,' I told a boy who had finally taken off his coat to join in. 'Left foot,' I said, picking mine off the floor and pointing in the direction to turn, 'That way.' He looked up, still confused. 'It's this one,' I said, tapping my bare foot on his trainer, and he smiled, shaking his head as my heart swelled with gladness.

As we moved through the class, I started thinking here was a room of teenagers who are at the bottom of the barrel in terms of who the yoga and so-called wellness industry is interested in targeting with its airy studios in affluent post-codes. In a way, capitalist wellness as it stands seems to serve those who are already reasonably 'well', or at least well off enough to pay for the privilege. And yet this practice may have actually been designed all along for young people like the teenagers I was meeting this evening. Indian guru Tirumalai Krishnamacharya, widely dubbed 'the father of modern yoga', devised Ashtanga Vinyasa – a vigorous method of postural yoga to build strength and stamina among his students who were, according to some historians, mostly young boys. Several years into my own relationship with yoga and when I was hooked on Ashtanga, I was distraught to read an article by the controversial cult leader Osho who went as far as to say women shouldn't practise Ashtanga because it would shrink their breasts and damage their wombs. I was so disturbed by what I read that I asked my Ashtanga teacher at the time what to do. Would I have to stop? I asked him. I didn't want to stop. Thankfully he suggested I ignore Osho and carry on as I was. Ashtanga was further popularized in the West in the 1940s by Pattabhi Jois – one of Krishnamacharya's students. Decades later it was *the* approach to yoga everyone seemed to be practising – including the likes of Madonna, Gwyneth Paltrow (and me).

The claim that Ashtanga was created for teenage boys has since been refuted by many, and the history of yoga's origins are notoriously hazy since it's so old, so who knows what's true? I don't think it matters. Ashtanga is harder to find as a method for practising yoga at studios these days, mostly I think because it has a reputation for being strict and following a set routine of postures. There are definitely dogmatic Ashtanga teachers out there; I've met many and not gone back to practise with them. That austere approach is not the way I teach either. I teach in a way that follows the traditional Ashtanga sequence as well as using the breath in a specific way because it works for me and I like to teach what I practise.

But I don't do everything by the rule book. I also sometimes skip poses in classes I teach when we only have one hour to practise, so that regular students can be introduced to more postures. I do this to keep the practice interesting but also because everyone is at various stages in their yoga journey. In drop-in classes, I adapt what I teach depending on who turns up. Everyone's bodies will respond to the postures differently; some may find something impossible to do earlier in the sequence whereas a posture that comes later might feel more accessible. I know this because I spent a long time in the same place in my own Ashtanga practice and it was only when I mixed things up a bit and started to practise postures that appear in later sequences that I discovered shapes my body responded to comfortably, whereas there are other postures that come earlier that I might never get the hang of simply because of the way my body (and mind) is made.

So I hope with this book I can help shed the unhelpful image Ashtanga seems to have developed over the years. It's sometimes considered 'too hard', 'too rigid', or 'boring' by modern yogis who want to be able to freestyle rather than follow a prescribed sequence. But it's none of those things if you don't want it to be. I would go as far as to say it's one of the most accessible ways of practising because everything is laid out for you. And I have proof that students enjoy the practice when I've taught classes without telling anyone what we're doing. They've often been surprised by how much they got out of the practice on discovering they were learning Ashtanga all along.

Ashtanga had its own heyday, which was still going strong when I discovered it in the late 1990s, and it has played a large part in what made yoga so popular in the Western world, which shows that it can help people from all walks of life.

The Ashtanga approach has since been rearranged and remixed to form many other approaches to practising by teachers in the West. Having more styles is useful in a way as it means there's more variety for people to find a way they like to practise. On the other hand, I sometimes wonder if yoga is losing something every time it gets repurposed.

Vinyasa Flow is arguably the most popular class taught all over the world from what I've seen on my travels. Vinyasa, as well as other styles like Rocket and Jivamukti, wouldn't exist without Ashtanga. That said, while the methods and vehicles through which postural yoga is practised have changed over the years, the philosophy to which it is attached remains the same. That's the bit that gives the postures a function and purpose. Although I've been fickle, explored and dabbled with many approaches to yoga, I've always returned to Ashtanga, particularly at times when the idea of practice has felt tough. I don't have to think about it and can just get on with it. For that reason, I think Ashtanga sometimes attracts many people who are restless, prone to anxiety and sometimes have more energy than they know what to do with. It's what drew me to it. There's so much detail to focus on – how you're moving your body, controlling the breath, where you're putting the gaze – that you simply have to stop thinking about anything other than what you're doing. It's an excellent approach for beginners because there is lots of repetition. With practice one can memorize and internalize the sequence so that eventually you can practise alone without having to rely on a teacher to guide you.

It made sense to me that Ashtanga would work for teenagers (given the confusing and transformative time they are having) whether it was designed for them or not. None of the boys in the North London community centre had practised yoga before, though some of them later told me they'd heard that yoga had something to do with feeling relaxed. I was heartened that so many of them took to it or were at least curious: keenly inhaling and reaching their arms up, exhaling, folding forward and jumping back into plank pose as we did the Sun Salutation sequences and moved through the other postures. The session was fun, as I had hoped, but it was also tiring. It was nothing like teaching the average class in a yoga studio. Everyone was squashed despite the large room because tables and chairs had to be pushed to the sides. There were zero frills: no mood lighting, no candles, incense or other tranquil enhancements. Our mats looked like they had seen a fair few workouts in their time and there were no comfy bolsters or blankets. But it felt honest in that room, and much like the gym where I went to my first yoga class. A lot of the boys were rowdy because I assume they thought what I was showing them was ridiculous. I thought the same thing in my first class. Yoga poses *are* ridiculous until you get used to them. But I kept them moving, held the space and eventually won most of them over. That is, until it came to the relaxation bit at the end. I asked them to lie down for Savasana (Corpse Pose) and to stay as still as they could. Some of them looked at me suspiciously. Who could blame them? But I continued.

'I'm going to turn the lights off for two minutes. Can we see if it's possible to be quiet and still?' I asked, sounding like a primary school teacher. 'It's just two minutes . . .' Nope. As soon as I flicked the switch, the room erupted with laughter. I turned the lights back on and we wrapped up. I thanked everyone for having me and rushed over to a corner to pull my trainers on. Belal and a few of the others came over to say thank you and that they felt calmer from the session. I was touched and pleased that it had worked and that they seemed to like me and my informal, 'come on everyone, let's give this a go' teaching style. I felt relieved but also couldn't wait to get out of there. It's tough when you're faced with scepticism and reluctance. As yoga teachers, when we're teaching the paying public we're not going to please them all, but one thing we're certain of is that they all want to be there. I walked back down the corridor to leave, telling myself the evening had gone well but with a sinking feeling that I might not have the stamina to return. The pay was barely liveable. I would earn £30 for what was essentially four hours of work including travel time.

Back outside, I noticed the knot in my stomach was back and my breath was getting shorter. I was too wound up to do anything sensible like take deep breaths. I realized I was feeling sorry for myself because I didn't feel valued. This charity work I did was the toughest but also the most life-affirming. It felt meaningful and I wanted to do it more, but it was draining and under-funded, which meant very little cash made it into the hands of the teachers. My income came mostly from covering drop-in classes in yoga studios and leisure centres and even that wasn't enough to get by. While I was lucky to come face to face with some lovely people who enjoyed my classes, the work itself was wearing me down. I found it draining to constantly meet new people from cover-teaching classes that weren't mine. I also felt that I was expected to lead exercise classes, which I tried very hard not to do because it didn't seem right in terms of how I practised yoga. Yet the pressure to do that was always on. I preferred teaching workshops, courses and my own regular classes so I could explain things more thoroughly and build relationships with people I would see again, but there wasn't enough of that work around. So I carried on with the work for the charity. Over time I found that I was most fulfilled working with marginalized – or deliberately silenced, as a charity worker friend of mine describes them – groups. But I didn't have a day job anymore. I'd long before walked out of my former life as a newspaper journalist and other salaried communications and PR jobs that followed. Gone were the days of payroll, and instead I was travelling every inch of London to teach as many classes as I could to make ends meet. I was constantly on tubes and trains collecting little bits of money that some teenagers might consider pocket money because I didn't have the reassurance of a monthly cash injection anymore.

This feeling of being undervalued had been brewing. I had started out a couple of years earlier as an assistant teacher for a charity that ran yoga classes for refugees. My voluntary role was to demonstrate poses at a mother-and-baby group while the lead teacher gave instructions. But I was plunged in at the deep end one week when the main teacher didn't turn up. I tried to get out of teaching because I've had a pathological fear of public speaking all my life and didn't want the spotlight. But the group's coordinator insisted, so I was forced to improvise. My chest tightened as I dragged a chair to the front of the room as slowly as I could, wondering what I was going to do. I hadn't signed up for this. I didn't want to be a yoga teacher, I had just come here to help out. It was my first time faced with a room of people waiting for me to show them what to do. I took the group through a series of simple breathing techniques and incorporated gentle movements that they could do seated in chairs. I made everything up as I went along but it did the trick. As I grew calmer, it became easier, more natural and I felt I had their trust. They loved it. I did too.

I was aware that many clients had caught several buses to attend. They came because yoga helped them sleep better, offered calm in the midst of uncertainty and helped them look inward. This is a big part of what the essence of yoga is meant to be: learning about and knowing yourself. What these women described sounded like genuine yoga in practice. Several months later, I asked the charity if I could have my own class. It was a group attended by Bengali and Somali women. They couldn't be further from the white Western stereotype of a fancy-pants yogini. We were crammed into a back room in an East London community space, over capacity which the centre manager thankfully turned a blind eye to because I refused to turn anyone away. That class was my favourite for a long time, and it was sometimes chaotic. Many of the women were mothers so we had snoozing babies in buggies, and a toddler or two running between the rows of arms and legs in Downward Facing Dog Pose. It was this keeping-it-real chaos that made me love that class even more.

Each week I was inspired by the women's commitment: hijabs off and salwar kameez billowing around their legs, some of them wore long skirts that restricted how wide they could step with their feet. It didn't matter. We never did anything worthy of posting to social media in those classes. Just plain old poses as they were intended to be – breathing and moving to a strong rhythm. But the popular narrative of flexible, crop-topped bodies in handstands on beaches so often sold in health magazines, on YouTube and other social media was never my reality either. My practice has been far sweatier and less elegant than that and my experience as a yoga teacher includes working with people over seventy, others with disabilities, those suffering with mental illnesses and in recovery from substance misuse (like me). This is why I'm so passionate about yoga being inclusive.

The women told me they liked my energetic classes and were always up for whatever I offered, bending forwards, sideways and jumping into positions (which is the Ashtanga way) when I pushed them. Sometimes they were easily distracted, other times fiercely focused. That's how it is with yoga.

My heart had found somewhere it was meant to be. But the charity's rules were that I had to teach that class as a volunteer for several months before I was eligible to get paid. This meant that teaching yoga to people in these circumstances turned out to be a huge financial strain – even though I was nourished by doing it. The hard fact was that I needed to earn a living. So I started adding classes in leisure centres to my schedule, which led to classes in ritzy yoga studios, and work with private clients soon followed. But sessions like the one with the teenage boys that November night became even harder to do because teaching more elsewhere meant that I was exhausted all the time. It's also emotionally demanding taking care of vulnerable groups, encouraging them to trust you and the practice. It's not lucrative. It was important work, but my stamina was waning because it was underpaid and there was no pastoral support. Charities like the one I worked for were making a valuable contribution, but it was just a massive shame that those working there weren't being looked after. I'd also been told – off the record – by an independent consultant tasked with writing an impact report about the charity that there were concerns about a lack of ethnic diversity among teachers leading classes. Money wasn't their only problem. Turning this over in my mind as I crossed the road towards the station, I felt sad. I had to admit that I'd probably never see those boys again or find out how they got here. Job satisfaction just wasn't enough to live on: I needed to pay the bills.

The Sun Salutation

I stand at the top of the mat, feeling stiff, achy and heavy. Big toes touching, heels apart. I lift all ten toes off the floor, spread them and place them back down. I stand in Samasthiti, Equal Standing Pose, (commonly known as Mountain Posture).

I pause.

Can I be bothered to practise now?

My body hurts.

Life hurts.

What's the point?

It's the afternoon and I usually do this in the morning. But I'm anxious and jumpy so I stick with it. Everything begins with the Sun Salutation – the backbone of all postural practice. Even when there's no time to practise, I always do this. Over and again until I am tired and feel I will be able to sit still. When I first learnt the Sun Salutation it reminded me of *Namaz* – the Muslim practice for performing prayer, which involves raising arms and bowing down. This familiarity, given my Muslim roots, gave me a fondness for this series of movements. I bring my palms together, thumbs to chest and quickly whisper the Ashtanga Yoga opening chant. Then, inhaling and reaching arms up, pressing palms together, I look at my thumbs, exhaling as I fold forwards and place palms flat on the floor.

Urgh, I'm tired, haven't had enough sleep and my brain feels tight.

I inhale, extend my hurting heart forward, then exhale and jump into a plank position. I lower my body down, hovering above the mat in Chaturanga Dandasana or Four-legged Stick Pose. Inhaling again, I roll over the toes and lift into Upward Facing Dog, exhaling into Downward Facing Dog Pose. I notice that I'm holding my breath. It's hard to breathe.

My hips are stuck. I feel the same way about life at the moment.

Still in Downward Facing Dog, I spread my fingers wide, shoulders away from the ears, tailbone to the sky, heels sinking towards the earth. I inhale one, exhale one. Inhale two, exhale two. I count five long jaggedy breaths like this. Then, inhaling, I jump feet to hands, lengthen forward and exhale to fold. Inhaling again, reaching arms up and exhale arms down, back to the Mountain.

I am solid as a mountain, I tell myself.

Firm as the earth.

A knot in my stomach tightens, telling me otherwise.

I must keep pushing through.

I start counting silently in Sanskrit, which sometimes helps block out the mental noise that never seems to stop. *Ekam* arms up, *dve* fold forward, *trini* lift heart, *chatvari* jump back and lower down. I keep going. My body's weight is starting to spread more evenly in my feet, the oil in my hips starting to loosen things. Soon my brain might catch up. I take five breaths in Downward Dog again. I'm tired and distracted.

Maybe I'm hungry, I should stop, a voice in my head says.

Keep going, another one suggests.

Okay then.

I continue, inhaling then reaching up, exhaling and folding forward. Now the breath feels like it's leading my movement. A lightness arrives in my body and my mind is narrowing its focus. The yoga is gaining momentum. This is what the physical part of the practice is for – preparing the body for meditation. I'm ready now.

Everything might turn out alright after all.

I jump feet to hands, and sit down, pulling my feet towards hips for Padmasana, Lotus Pose. I press the index fingers and thumbs of each hand together and sit, eyes closed. The thoughts in my head come into view – still tangled. I focus on the Third Eye in the middle of the forehead above the eyebrows. The Third Eye is believed to be the seat of all wisdom, the place where our intuition rests. I need some of that now, more than ever. Twenty-five slow breaths, filling me up and leaving me empty. Finally, I open my eyes. That's better. I'm calmer, no longer imprisoned in a submarine of 'What am I doing with my life?' thoughts.

Practising yoga teaches you how simple life can be. It nudges you towards what's right in front of you – going inward instead of looking outward, and being in the moment. If you concentrate, it's possible to become immersed within it and reframe your perspective.

It makes me realize how easily I get caught up in planning and controlling my life. When I step back, I can see that it's often my own thoughts that are causing me problems. Yoga helps me disidentify with all those thought patterns that seem so solid, so real, so identity-defining. The thoughts that tell me I'm not loveable, not good enough, have failed at life. Left untended, they get bigger, louder and more repetitive until I believe them all, which leaves me in a tangle of self-absorbed pain. When I practise, I have an opportunity to notice that I am not my thoughts and I almost always recognize I have fewer problems than I believed.

Watching the breath, listening to its sound, and observing the body fully takes effort, so it's a constant juggle to find balance between effort and ease. When we start practising yoga it may seem impossible to switch the mind stuff off, but if you focus on what you're doing, slowly it becomes conceivable that you can unplug and put your attention on your body and breath alone. The key thing is to focus the mind upon the breath with such unwavering attention that the thoughts cease to be – even if for the briefest of moments. It takes practice, and practice makes us stronger. It's this transformative aspect of yoga that I discover anew every single time I get on my mat. The hardest thing is stepping onto it. First thing in the morning every excuse creeps in:

I haven't slept enough.

I'm depressed.

My head hurts.

I can't be bothered.

I hate my body.

There's no time.

Social media is killing the spirit of yoga.

And so it goes on.

Even decades after I went to my first yoga class there are days I don't want to practise, and I have to convince myself of what usually happens when I do: things shift and life becomes more bearable. I wake up to what's real and what's not. That's what meditation is for: being aware of what is. Doing the physical poses means looking at the mind and body as they are – not as I'd like them to be. Over time, this practice of observing helps me think and feel things more clearly. It can also help me accept things as they are. It isn't easy, but any of us can practise if we're willing to do the work. You just need to start. There's no need for a plant-based diet if you don't want that, and expensive equipment, fancy active wear and meditation-style playlists aren't obligatory either. These 'prerequisites' are all parts of what I call the wellness myth. You don't even need to love or accept yourself. I didn't at the beginning. I was filled with fear and self-loathing so there's definitely no need to feel the good vibes only. It helps if you're interested in learning to meditate in order to move towards higher states of consciousness because that's what real yoga is meant to be. It was never intended to be a mindfulness app or stop gap squeezed into a lunch break. Which is why what's happened to yoga in recent years is so tragic.

CHAPTER 2

On the Mat, 1996

While I was left disillusioned by yoga soon after I started teaching, it hadn't always been like that. The very first time I discovered yoga was quite different. My mum took me to a class when I was sixteen and I didn't even want to go. Refusing to take no for an answer, Mum shoved me in her car and drove us to a Hatha Yoga class at the local YMCA in East London in the spring of 1996. She had been going to the weekly class alone for a while and was tired of me moping in my bedroom. I remember the YMCA fondly; it was a large but unassuming building opposite the more opulent-looking Town Hall that stood behind a fountain and plush green lawn. We were cutting it fine with time, so Mum swerved into the car park out front and we were inside before I had time to catch up with what was going on.

We walked into a frenzy of activity: phones ringing, efficient-looking staff running in and out of doorways, a friendly receptionist, a queue growing at the canteen. It was a bustling spot but also relaxed with a strong feeling of a community that reflected the people who lived in the area. The kind of place that sadly seems rare to find these days. The YMCA's main operation was its attached accommodation, which offered supported housing for vulnerable and homeless people, others living with mental illness and learning disabilities or those recovering from substance misuse. As we weaved towards the sports hall where the class was due to take place, I started feeling nervous, wondering if it was too late to turn back. I didn't want to do this anymore, but Mum was marching ahead. The further away she went, the more reluctant I felt. We were going into the unknown, and I was trying not to get worked up but couldn't help feeling scared. I knew I would feel awkward in the class and everyone would stare because I wouldn't know what to do. I couldn't go through with it. *Maybe Mum's forgotten where it is, and we can go home*, I thought. I hoped.

'It's in here. Come on,' Mum called urgently. 'It'll be starting in a minute.'

It was too late to turn back now. I gave up and followed her inside. The room was massive, overwhelming and mostly empty. It looked like a school hall with basketball nets installed and yellow and white markings for other sports on the floor. A couple of people had settled on their mats already, eyes closed, lying down, feet on the floor, knees pointing to the ceiling, breathing into their hands on bellies. They looked comfortable. I wasn't. The idea of having to touch my stomach felt awful. This didn't look good at all. I shouldn't have agreed to come.

My mum had brought me to the class because I'd become an anxious teenager and had started to restrict what I ate. I thought that I had been doing a clever job of hiding it for a long time. Mum always seemed convinced when I lied and told her I'd already eaten when she offered to make me something, but I found out later she had been worrying for a while and trying to work out what to do. I was a stubborn and argumentative teenager so she wasn't going to have an easy job. The biggest challenge I faced was dinner, which we ate together, so I had to become an expert at tipping as much of my plate as I could onto kitchen paper laid out on my lap to throw away when my mum wasn't looking. I had a bad relationship with my body or at least felt disconnected from it. I felt clumsy inside it. I wanted my body to shrink because I didn't know what to do with it. I hated being noticed when I walked into a room full of people because I felt an intense paranoia that everyone was looking at me all the time. Eating disorders are not rational illnesses. It doesn't matter how smart or clever you are or whether you know loads about nutrition and healthy eating, as I did; when the disease has you in its grip there's no obvious way out. This is why it's unhelpful that these disorders get medicalized too often as physical problems. It's understandable with anorexia to a degree, where extreme weight loss becomes an issue, but I know from experience that putting on weight doesn't get rid of the problem that caused it in the first place. The UK charity Mind suggests that anorexia is linked to low self-esteem, negative self-image and feelings of intense distress.[1] The illness was once said to be the biggest killer of all the psychiatric disorders, particularly during adolescence. Of those surviving, 46 per cent recover, whereas 33 per cent improve and 20 per cent remain chronically ill.[2] But at that time eating disorders were not talked about openly so I wasn't aware that there were names for what I had started to do.

I wanted to take up as little space in the world as possible. Be smaller, invisible, disappear – for reasons I didn't know. I had been subjected to a few thoughtless comments by some pupils at secondary school about being chubby but nothing that would have disturbed a level-headed child or resulted in such an extreme response. It felt as though my head and body had rejected each other and were bobbing about in space, refusing to be friends. This is why I hadn't wanted to go to that first yoga class with my mum.

'Why don't you come with me this week?' she'd suggested earlier that day, her face hovering by my bedroom door. 'Don't fancy it,' I said from where I was sitting under a dreamcatcher on my bed. I was trying to make sense of *King Lear*, one of my college texts, but finding it impossible to concentrate. Why was Cordelia so awful? was the current question bugging me. I hadn't eaten since a few mouthfuls of rice and daal the night before, which was likely to have been why I couldn't focus.

'It'll do you good,' she persisted. I shook my head. I was aware that my mum seemed to be a fan of this yoga thing I had never heard of but it didn't sound good to me. 'I'll look stupid and I haven't got anything to wear,' I told her, going back to my book to indicate it was time for her to leave.

'Whack on a pair of trackies, and be downstairs in half an hour,' she said and disappeared from the doorway. I looked at the poster of Malcolm X on the opposite wall and my hungry stomach inflated with dread.

It's fair to say there wasn't much joy in my life at that time. There wasn't any space for it, which was a strange turn of events because I had been a happy and carefree child. By the time I was a teenager, worrying about everything – my body, exams, what others thought of me, the future – was my base-line mood. The less I ate, the more I thought about food. This obsession left little room to think about anything else, which is why I struggled with studying for long periods and drifted away from friendships. I kept a mental note of everything I ate and how many calories were in it. Calorie obsession is a punishing trap, but the longer I could go without food the more I felt like I was winning. I was a new vegetarian, which

I had chosen to be for ethical reasons. I had become preoccupied with animal welfare when I was ten and demanded to go veggie back then but Mum refused and said I would have to wait until I was sixteen. That's when vegetarianism became a convenient way to restrict my diet. But I was also always hungry and longed for the day that I wouldn't be. It started in my final year at an all-girls secondary school when I got fed up with my changing body. I didn't want puberty, I didn't want peer-pressure and judgement. I felt stifled. In a way my behaviour was less about avoiding a fat body and more about evading a female one. I didn't want breasts and I resented my periods. They became erratic and eventually stopped for several years, which felt like a mark of success because my dietary controls were obviously working. Without knowing it I was preserving my body to stay as a child because I wasn't ready to become a woman. I didn't feel like I ever would be.

In my eyes my mum was dazzling in both image and presence. She was glamorous and represented what a woman was supposed to be. I adored her, looked up to her and yet knew I would never be like her. I didn't feel like a woman, and part of me didn't want to be one.

There's no obvious reason why my disordered eating took hold. My mum had never been on a diet and I hadn't ever heard her say anything negative about her own body shape. She cooked everything from scratch and brown bread, wholegrain rice and homemade flapjacks were staples in our home. I developed healthy tastes and didn't care about sweets. An eating disorder shouldn't have happened. My parents had split up and got back together several times when I was very young but I didn't think that had anything to do with it. I saw my dad regularly as a child for a while but when I was nine he vanished without explanation. Until that point, he would pick me up and half-heartedly take me out to do something that both of us couldn't wait to be over. He once took me to a toy shop and said I could have anything I wanted. I picked a police car that I could drive around the communal gardens outside the flat where I lived with my mum. He told me that it wasn't appropriate for girls and got me a giant My Little Pony castle instead. It was a pink monstrosity that ended up in a charity shop. I spent the rest of my childhood believing my dad clearly didn't understand me and wondering why he stopped coming to visit.

Aside from the confusion around his disappearance, I was a happy child and loved primary school. I was popular, had lots of friends and endless energy that saw me bouncing around the playground every break time, playing any game that involved running.

Secondary school by contrast was hard. Beauty standards had been set, fashion and skirt lengths were remorselessly critiqued, and popularity endlessly contested. Rumours would fly around about who had started their periods, who had almost had sex or gone all the way. Coming from a Muslim home meant that I wasn't going to be joining in any of these teen rites of passage. I was a late bloomer when it came to puberty and, in such a competitive environment, self-consciousness kicked in. I would look at the popular girls with their good looks and up-to-date wardrobes and wonder what life must be like being so perfect. Mum wouldn't let me wear make-up – it was against the school rules but not wearing it meant that I felt ugly compared with other girls who modelled themselves on Bollywood film stars, dyed their hair with blonde highlights and were queens of flicky eye make-up. It felt like everyone around me was progressing and I was being left behind. After being the centre of attention at primary school, I was now a lone wolf, drifting in and out of circles of friends but not belonging to any of them. Some girls said I was fat; I wasn't but I believed them. Muslim girls criticized me because I wore ankle socks in summer with bare legs, didn't wear a headscarf and my mum wouldn't let me fast during Ramzaan (what we Pakistanis call Ramadan).

'Children shouldn't keep *rozeh* [fasts],' she would say. 'But all the other girls are doing it,' I'd argue. 'No,' she would push back, and that was that. Every year it was the same. She wouldn't budge.

When I got to year ten, I was made a prefect. I was surprised my teachers believed I had the leadership qualities for the job. The role gave me some confidence for a while. I started bending the rules; I wore jewellery that wasn't allowed, untucked my shirt and let younger kids I felt sorry for off detention. I utilized the prefect power I had by trying to change the way that things were run. The first act of civil disobedience I initiated was against our school uniform. We were forced to wear skirts, and I felt that we should have the choice to wear trousers if we wanted. One lunchtime I persuaded a small group of girls to wear their PE kits for a demonstration in the playground. The deputy headteacher came running out within ten minutes. We never did get to wear the trousers. It was soon after that food became a problem. Disorder: I seemed to enjoy creating it. It swirled around me and maybe that's because I felt it inside. Mum said I had a habit of self-sabotaging, meaning that I got in the way of good things happening for me. I wasn't sure what she was talking about and didn't agree.

Before trying yoga on me, my mum intervened by taking me to the doctor after she clocked my dinner was going in the bin. The doctor told her I wasn't underweight and that she shouldn't worry. Mum didn't listen and persuaded me to put on weight. I refused but my mum persevered. The pressure piled up, and I gave in. I started forcing myself to eat giant plates of food at home that my stomach didn't know what to do with. Fullness was impossible to bear but I kept going just to get my mum off my back. I thought I could return to starving when she stopped paying so much attention to me. I wasn't smart enough to realize that my mum was never going to lose interest in her child.

Soon I was cramming chocolate bars into my mouth on the way home from school even when I wasn't hungry. I ate resentfully and in a disassociated way, hardly aware of the food going into my mouth, which was similar to the numbness I had felt when I was restricting my intake. Over time, this anxious way of eating developed into secret binges in my bedroom. I felt ashamed for eating as much as I was but I couldn't seem to stop. After months of restricting food, I felt I had lost control, which made me despise my body more. I gained a little weight but by the time I was in sixth form college I'd discovered how to make myself sick. I didn't know what bulimia was but I rationalized that it might help reverse the weight I had gained. It didn't work. Instead, I ended up with a puffy face, swollen throat and permanently sore stomach. My teeth started to crumble and in some cases fall out because that's what stomach acid (which isn't meant to be in your mouth) does to them. I still hated my body and I hated being sick, but I was possessed by a demon forcing me to its will. I felt I had no choice. I had a mental illness but was in denial. Bulimia is a hidden illness that's still not as understood as it could be. It involves an obsession of the body, a fixation on food, both of which are distractions from a bigger problem that the sufferer can't identify. 'About three quarters of patients with anorexia and more than half of all patients with bulimia, are bewildered by their emotional feelings and have great difficulty describing them,' Bessel Van Der

Kolk writes in *The Body Keeps the Score*.[3] There's even a word for it: alexithymia, which is when a person struggles to identify and express how they feel. That's how it was for me. For years I thought I wanted to be thin but in truth my eating disorders were just cover-ups for avoiding my feelings.

Being sick sucks the life out of you because of the toll it takes on the body but also having to be three steps ahead of everything with all the plotting, planning and lying that comes with it, and constant cleaning and bleaching of the toilet so no one finds out. I'd crawl into bed after a heavy session of throwing up, exhausted. I would spend hours searching online for ways I could stop eating again. I trawled pro-anorexia forums online for tips on how to reverse my behaviour and felt worse because no one talked about being sick there. I looked up to anorexics because they had the discipline I was so desperate for and wanted back. Of course, I now know better and those with anorexia feel as trapped and enslaved as I did. The difference was that what I was doing was messy and out of control. It felt like I was the only person in the world going through this, and I was doing this terrible secret thing because I didn't hear many stories about kids having food problems, least of all Pakistani girls like me. I was clearly a freak as I suspected.

I can't imagine what it was like for my poor mum living with someone determined to destroy herself, least of all her child. We went back to the same doctor and Mum demanded that I be referred to an eating-disorder service. I went through several Cognitive Behavioural Therapists as an outpatient at a hospital where the toilets had locks on the outside and every room I went into smelled of boiled potatoes. I felt sorry for the in-patients because being forced to keep food in my body when I had an urgent need to get rid of it all the time sounded impossible. The first CBT therapist I was assigned decided that I would outgrow what she suggested was a teenage phase. Another said she couldn't work with me because I failed to do the homework, which involved keeping a food diary and identifying the very thing I was avoiding – my feelings – every time I ate. The final therapist turned me away because she didn't think I wanted to get better. She wasn't wrong. My mum wasn't happy that the hospital discharged me but I was glad therapy was over. I didn't like CBT. Every therapist I met sounded like they were reading from a textbook rather than talking to me as the uniquely messed-up person I believed I was. I could see through it. I wasn't like the case studies they talked about; I was different. Psychology wasn't a new subject to me. Mum, a former primary school teacher, had been doing a Master's degree in educational psychology at the time. Our bookshelves at home were filled with books on psychology, positive thinking and spirituality so I believed I knew everything there was to know about emotional wellbeing – and I wasn't interested in any of it. Mum would encourage me to come up with affirmations and would write them out in her wide school-teacher handwriting for me to stick on my bedroom wall. I humoured her but couldn't see what good they were going to do. I wasn't going to be easy to help.

Magical Properties

After everything she had already tried, my mum's suggestion of yoga was an attempt to drag me out of my bedroom (and the bathroom) to steer me towards a more level-headed path where I might discover some tools that empowered me to change. I wouldn't have to rely on a therapist I didn't believe in and could find my way on my own terms. At least that had been my mum's thinking. Around the time I went to that first yoga class at the YMCA I had been studying art as one of my

A-levels. When I wasn't in bed recovering from being sick, I would paint. Smearing oil paint on giant canvases in my bedroom was the only thing that diverted my attention from obsessing over food. Painting gave me a reprieve from my thoughts; making shapes offered moments of peace. It didn't matter to me that I wasn't any good at drawing; those solitary hours of absorbed concentration became a comfort, an escape from the cage of misery I had trapped myself in.

All in all, yoga was Mum's final attempt to get me out of my head, into my body and perhaps through the practice, find a way to connect the two. It was something that had worked for her. She'd become interested in yoga for what she said had felt like magical properties, when she was at secondary school. Her form tutor taught Transcendental Meditation after taking the morning register and encouraged her to explore yoga. Mum is the eldest child of her generation in her family, and she and her five siblings weren't allowed to watch much TV so she found other hobbies: sewing, drawing, writing stories and learning yoga poses. Years later after her marriage was over, Mum returned to yoga while exploring Zen meditation. I was three at the time and we were living together in a women's refuge. Mum called it The Roundhouse after the circular window in the front door. We lived in one room with a double bed, sofa and kettle for nine months until a council flat became available. For me, living in The Roundhouse was an adventure because my mum presented it to me that way, but looking back, it must have been a hard time for her. Yoga made her feel grounded and helped her to discover who she was again. Despite my initial resistance, many years later, I can see why she turned to it as a way to find stability in her otherwise uncertain life.

* * *

The lights were bright for that hour of yoga in the YMCA hall. There were about twelve of us and the gender split of men and women was relatively equal. We were all wearing tracksuits and there weren't any statues of Hindu gods or Om symbols in sight. There were no vegan brunch deals on offer, power smoothies or turmeric lattes for sale. There wasn't even any music.

Our instructor, Davina, was short with a dark brown bob haircut and could have been any age. I guessed she might be forty. She had a deep slightly orange tan, like a strong mug of builder's brew, and was wearing white linen trousers and a floaty white tunic shirt. She looked different to the rest of us – smarter, settled in her skin and confident but not in an intimidating way. She talked us through what I would now describe as a gentle beginner-friendly class. There was no fuss or elaborate choreography, and the postures weren't as scary as I'd imagined they would be. She didn't explain much about what yoga was or why we might be doing it. She didn't use the Sanskrit names of the poses either, and instead there was a simplicity and sincerity in the way she offered the practice to us. Davina wasn't overselling yoga or performing a role, she didn't make jokes or try to be our friend. I didn't get the sense that she was trying to make us like her or look up to her either. She seemed deeply at ease within herself, explaining what to do and coming from a place that looked very sure about what yoga did for her in her life. I liked that quiet confidence I saw. Did she get it from yoga, I wondered?

I was uncomfortable for the first ten minutes of class and looked around the room to check no one was laughing at me. I felt foolish in Triangle Pose, straining to reach my right arm down the right leg and wonkily stretching my left arm into the air. I felt awkward standing on one leg in a wobbling Tree Pose. But after a while and without any ceremony, I mentally dropped into what we were doing. For the first time in years – perhaps ever – I felt that I was getting a sense of stepping out of my head and truly experiencing my body in a non-competitive way. A shift took place as I was starting to focus less on what my body looked like and was discovering what it could do.

Thinking back to that class, it's astonishing that I was so open to it, considering the battleground my body had been. The body I was hiding in loose combat trousers and baggy sweatshirts, the one I wasn't feeding properly. Yoga focused awareness on my body, which, given the way my head was inclined, could have set me up for self-criticism – I'm not bendy enough, not strong enough, too wobbly – but it didn't. Somehow the practice was shifting focus away from the aesthetics of my body and onto function and moving in strange new ways. Something powerful was happening that didn't make sense, but it felt good. At the end of the class we laid down in Savasana. It was the first time I'd ever done it and I felt an entirely new lightness and sense of ease wash over my body. My mind was calm. I listened to Davina talk us through a relaxation process. I felt self-contained and glacially still. It might have been the first time I'd ever felt like that. The usual thoughts buzzing and ricocheting around my mind started to slow down. My body felt heavier as we lay there, sinking into the mat, and yet there was a new openness and weightlessness in my chest; a feeling as if I was hovering an inch above the floor. I felt pleasantly dissociated from my brain and content in my body. It was an unfamiliar yet comforting sensation. Those usual thoughts:

I hate my stomach . . .

I'm too fat . . .

How many calories have I eaten today?

Suddenly I noticed they weren't there. Instead, there was a

new sensation where my entire body was still and relaxed, only the breath moving. I focused on that natural movement. *Easy breath coming in, easy breath going out.* I felt completely at peace, like I'd drifted into a transcendental reality, and didn't want it to end. It sounds dramatic because it was. I don't know how long we were lying there, I lost track of time. The class was only an hour so it couldn't have been long, but I felt like I'd been resting like that for weeks. As we walked out, Mum told me I definitely had to go back the following week. 'I'm not taking no for an answer,' she said. 'I mean it, Nadi, you look two inches taller and so serene! How do you feel?'

I couldn't tell. I admitted that I felt kind of floaty, and like something cosmic had happened inside me that I couldn't describe. 'I feel relaxed, I think. It was good,' I said. 'I told you it would work,' Mum said, looking pleased with herself. We both started laughing at the same time at the strange magic in the air, and got into the car. I felt like I had experienced a psychic change, a permanent shift that meant I would never be the same again. Either that or I was under a spell. My brain was quieter, less tight. What had happened to me there? I wondered. The only way I'd find out would be to return. And we did for many weeks and months. Soon I started exploring yoga on my own, seeking out other teachers and classes to try. It became a hobby and a new obsession. Pretty much everywhere I've travelled across the world in the decades since that first class, my yoga mat has gone with me. Yoga has been there, a constant in my life. There have been times I have drifted away from it but I have somehow found myself returning to it even when I haven't been sure why. I've just always known that it will help because that first experience was so powerful. So that's how I made friends with yoga, or it became friends with me, and like many a great friendship, we've also fallen out at times.

CHAPTER 3

Everything Hurts

I often wish my experience with yoga had been simpler. I would love to say that yoga saved me instantly and life has been filled with clear skies and beautiful sunsets ever since we met. But it was more complex than that. While yoga has supported me more than I can probably convey, it wasn't the only thing that helped when life was hard to navigate. My yoga journey isn't one of triumph over tragedy. It has been more intricate than that because I had a dysfunctional relationship with food and my body when I was first introduced to yoga and it didn't solve the problem. In fact, while I continued to explore yoga, my disorder got progressively worse for a while. I'm not sure why it went like that. It could have been because I was quite young when I discovered the practice and didn't have the emotional skills to connect the problem – my disorder – with yoga and allow it to form a bigger part of the solution towards recovery.

Though I love yoga there have been many occasions I've had arguments with it and walked out on it too. Those were times when the yoga spell seemed to break and the practice appeared to stop working. This was when emotional disturbances pulled me away like break-ups, work stresses and other general hazards of being a human trying to make sense of life. I gave up practising at some of those times by accident – yoga just slipped away. At other times, I didn't practise because as yoga became more popular and seen as something that went along with a healthy lifestyle I realized that I wasn't who a yoga person was meant to be. That person was calm, looked after their body and generally had their life in order – definitely not me.

Although I started noticing problems with yoga again when I started teaching, the truth is that for a long time, *I* might have been the problem. There were many years that yoga and I spent face down on the floor and where I couldn't move forward. I felt let down by yoga at those times too, but of course it wasn't yoga's fault. The truth is I hadn't given the practice a chance. Until slowly I did. It's this slipping and sliding backwards and forwards rather than an upward curve that I think has taught me most about yoga since the practice and I first met decades ago. I have now accepted that the twists and turns and wounds of the past have made my practice deeper simply by forcing me to think about it and question what it all means as the years have gone by. I doubt this would have happened if life had been plain sailing since that first class at the YMCA.

This isn't meant to be a sob story, but it is a reality check. There have been plenty of good times in my life, for which I am grateful. And there have been excruciating periods where I struggled and couldn't see an end to the pain. Yoga didn't always offer solutions but now I look back it makes me wonder how much harder everything would have been if I hadn't discovered the practice even if at those times I lost faith in it for a short while. So I think it's important to talk about some of the difficult stuff that drew me closer to yoga but that also pulled me away from it. I think it's essential to look at this because when life's going well it's so much easier to practise; it's when we're struggling that we need it most and when, in my experience, it is harder to do. It's also when the going gets tough that I've gained my biggest insights in life and I'll be sharing some of them in this book. I'll do my best to tell you how I have worked through some of the hard times both with and without my practice and how I have finally made peace with yoga in ways that have changed my life. My approach to the practice now is also different to the way I applied it to my life in the past, which I think feels honest. I say this because my life's been a series of beginnings, endings (and glorious bits in between). The biggest gift was staying alive, even when I thought I didn't know how to. I've changed, so my practice has had to change too. So, before we go on, it's worth telling you a bit more about how I got here.

I was born in Hackney, East London in 1980. After my parents split up for good, my mum and I lived in a two-bed flat and she studied to become a primary school teacher so that we could take summer holidays together. Having me at twenty-one while she was still so young gave her the strength to leave her marriage and build a new life for herself. I was too young to appreciate that as a child and didn't know that our life was different to anyone else's, but it was. I might have missed out on having siblings but I was there for so many significant milestones in my mum's life. I idolized her. We were a team and did everything together. I would hang out with her mates in the university canteen when she was in lectures, and I sat in the back seat of the car, reading books and making up poems while Mum took driving lessons up front. (It was the 1980s and there were fewer health and safety rules!) I was content and happy.

Mum took me to Pakistan (her birthplace) when I was eight, which is still one of the happiest periods of my life. It was a time of freedom, of discovery and having space to express myself. I remember running, sandals off, barefoot through the heavy monsoon rain and splashing around in Tarbela Dam, the world's largest dam that runs along the Indus River. It was a time of joy and safety, where I was free to roam the local villages with my new friends without the watchful eye of adults.

Mum and I stayed for five months, and she had been considering a fresh start there with me. I sometimes think about how my life would have been if we'd stayed. Would it have been better, worse or just different? It wasn't meant to be. My dad arrived on my birthday and pleaded with my mum to come back. We returned to live with him in London and I realized I had forgotten how to speak English. It had disappeared. The words were there in my nine-year-old head but I couldn't get them out. I had been speaking Urdu for so long I was out of practice. It may have been a silent protest about being forced to leave a place I loved. Maybe I was fed up with my dad, whose presence seemed to disrupt any equilibrium we had found, meaning we had to move all the time whether we were going to live with him or leaving to get away. Somehow, part of me was refusing to come home. Luckily my English returned when I settled back in school, but my parent's reunion didn't last and we left again to live at the same rented flat we had been in before. Later that year, my dad stopped his weekly visits to see me. It was an abrupt end and I didn't understand. I thought it was because he didn't like me. That had to be the case because in my child's mind I couldn't find another explanation for such rejection. When I was a teenager, my mum reminded me that I could get in touch with my dad if I wanted to. She had never tried to turn me against him and suggested it would be best for me to confront that early abandonment. But I wasn't interested in my dad if he wasn't interested in me. I batted my mum's idea away at around the same time I turned my back on food.

I thought that if I got top grades it would fill an inner void I seemed to have and I would be happy. I did and I wasn't. Eating disorders are almost always linked with an obsessive need to control things, but it still isn't clear to me what I was trying to control – my own happiness maybe. By the time I arrived at university I was going to yoga classes several nights a week with different teachers at plush-looking studios (there weren't many of them in London at the time, but they were all an upgrade from the YMCA). I chose high-energy classes that pushed my body and made me sweat – this didn't stop my bulimia but curbed the number of times I was making myself sick so I kept at it.

I couldn't settle in at university and felt lost. I had chosen to do an obscure degree in South Asian Studies at The University of London's SOAS (School of Oriental and African Studies) perhaps as a way to learn more about my ancestry and identity to help find my place in the world. Getting to study Indian cinema felt like a cheeky thrill (I grew up around family members obsessed with Bollywood). But real life felt like hard work so I was drawn to abstract ideas, living in the romantic fairy tales of the movies and learning about the past. I was captivated by the Urdu literature classes. I learnt about colonialism and South Asian politics through the poetry of Muhammad Iqbal and Faiz Ahmed Faiz. I couldn't get enough of Saadat Hasan Manto's stories about the partition of India, but struggled to make sense of Farsi, which I really wanted to learn. In history lectures I learnt about the Upanishads and

Vedas – ancient sacred texts containing hymns and philosophy about the natural order of the world. These important texts pre-date all modern religions in India and contain the first mentions of yoga. I found the descriptions of early rituals and sacrificial fire ceremonies fascinating to begin with, but this part of history was new to me and soon got too confusing to follow because my concentration was still so poor.

I didn't drink and found it hard to make friends, so yoga was my refuge even though it was starting to feel like a burden too. I became hooked on dynamic classes and eventually found Ashtanga. It was often taught by strict teachers, which resulted in me becoming militant about practising as often as I could. If I had to miss a class due to lectures or a coursework deadline I felt like I'd let myself down. It wasn't a healthy relationship as yoga had become another stick to beat myself with. My renewed obsession with it squeezed all the early joy I had experienced at that first class. I wasn't sure if I still loved yoga but I was driven to stay close to it. I started volunteering at a posh new yoga studio in 2000 that had opened its doors just months earlier. My hope was that it would help me get closer to yoga and improve my relationship with it. It also gave me access to free classes, which helped on a student budget. The narrative around yoga back then was that it was a class that was good for your body and mind and had a spiritual side to it. I didn't know what this meant and, with all the lostness and emptiness I felt, I thought it was probably time to find out. But I didn't know where to start. None of the teachers talked much about how to access the spiritual side of things in the classes I went to and I didn't have the confidence to ask.

Volunteering at the studio gave me the opportunity to try a range of yoga styles. Still binging and purging and with a big appetite for practising in a strong way, it was at that studio I discovered Ashtanga. Not long after that I had a chance meeting with the late Pattabhi Jois, credited with popularizing Ashtanga yoga in the West, on his last visit to London. I roped my mum into coming to the studio at the last minute to make a giant pot of chai for Jois' visit because I was the only person in the building who knew someone that could. It was at that studio in 2000 that I first became aware that yoga was becoming popular in a way it hadn't been when I started practising. More people were talking about it, celebrities were doing it, features were appearing in magazines, and it was losing its dusty back-door image. This pleased me because it meant more opportunities to find classes. I was too wrapped up in my own troubles to question anything at that point. It never crossed my mind that in years to come yoga would become the global industry it is today.

From Lahore with Love

My relationship with Ashtanga grew deeper while I was at university but the classes remained joyless exercise routines that I could just about get to the end of since I was turning up after making myself sick the night before. There wasn't anything magical happening on my mat during that time but I thought if I kept pushing I might break through and find the jigsaw piece that was missing in my life. I might even have a spiritual experience if that's what yoga was really all about. This depressive period coincided with falling unexpectedly in love for the first time. I fell hard and fast and it was terrifying. Suddenly I was flooded with a load of new feelings that I didn't know what to do with. I hadn't fancied many people at school and because boyfriends were off limits,

I didn't have any experience of attraction or infatuation, which is what this was.

The object of my desire was a foreign student in my Urdu poetry class. She was from Lahore in Pakistan, a place I romanticized because it's where my grandparents lived after they got married and where my mum was born. We spent all of our free time in between classes together. We would walk through Bloomsbury and marvel at the poetry in the autumn leaves and crisp air in Russell Square. We would meet in the library, though I never got any work done because I couldn't stop looking at her. Being with her made me feel sick with excitement and fear about what was developing between us, and yet I couldn't bear us being apart. I hated what was happening to me and I was scared because I didn't want to be gay but it looked like I was. I didn't have any gay friends at the time and certainly none that were Muslim. I didn't think it was possible to reconcile those two things. I started rejecting the faith I was born into because it felt like the only way.

The Lahori knew I was besotted and enjoyed flirting with me, so I refused to see that my feelings were unrequited. She would leave handwritten verses by the poets Rilke, Rumi and Hafiz in my exercise books that I would analyze for days, searching for hidden clues to what she might be telling me. She came to stay over at home, where I was still living with my mum, and we lay in bed holding hands, electricity shooting up my legs under the covers. I was so seduced by her charm that I walked out on the first big love of my life: yoga. My mum didn't like the influence she was having and tried to steer me back towards the practice but I didn't need it anymore.

In our final year I told the Lahori that I might be gay. It was my clumsy way of opening up and hoping that this would mean we could be together, however blasphemous that might be. We were sitting on the steps outside the university on a cold afternoon, the sun lighting up her golden face. 'I always knew,' she said, gazing dreamily over my shoulder. She didn't talk to me much after that. I was confused. I'd destroyed the mirage between us by telling the truth. It was devastating and derailed my studies for the rest of the term. I just about scraped through my end-of-year exams and couldn't wait to get out of the university building and close that chapter of my life. I still believed I was gay and I came out to my mum. Mum listened, nodded and accepted what I was telling her. But knowing my mum as I do now, she would have had a million things running through her mind – chiefly concern that I was making a life choice that wouldn't be easy.

* * *

Once I'd finished university, I got a job working for a curator of spoken word events and moved into a bedsit in North London. I threw myself into the gay scene, which involved going to as many clubs as I could find. I went to my first Pride and loved it. I didn't feel loud or proud or political about my sexuality at that point because I was still working all that out. But I liked seeing people who were proud and it made me feel at home. I knew this new feeling wasn't just about the flags and rainbows and dancing in the street, though I found a huge sense of freedom in all of those things. Pride was about self-expression, identity and having the space to explore who I was. It was about acceptance and having somewhere to belong. I had found my community and didn't want to leave.

I was twenty-two when I stumbled into my first relationship. I first met – let's call her Z – in a basement drag bar in Soho the night I had my first drink. Still new to being out of the closet, I quickly noticed I'd overlooked the dress code. Most of the women in the room were wearing costume moustaches, suits, shirts and braces. I'd turned up in jeans and a green T-shirt with 'Wild Bird' written across it. I leaned against a wall by the toilets, clutching a Smirnoff Ice that I couldn't bear the taste of. It didn't take long before Z spotted me. She was ten years older than me and looked like an old punk rocker. She smelled dangerous: a heady mix of fags, leather and stolen perfume. Z embodied everything I wasn't and wanted to be: someone who had lived a full life and had the scars to prove it. She also had an eight-year heroin habit, which I was yet to discover. That familiar knot that lived in my stomach flared up, telling me I should beware, but after the rejection of the Lahori, being desired was hard to resist.

The welfare benefits Z claimed on grounds that she wasn't fit to work didn't cover the drugs she needed so she drank. Vodka was cheaper – or free on days she stole it. I started shoplifting booze too. I felt terrible every time I did it but I didn't stop because I got Z's approval when I did. A non-smoker until then, I started smoking weed with Z, and given that I was the one with the job, I paid for most of it. Z was angry when she'd been drinking and even violent to me. I had a black eye the first time I met Z's parents. 'Oh my God, they're going to know it was me,' she kept saying for what felt like the entire train journey. I stared blankly out of the window as London rooftops flashed by and turned into Essex countryside. We told them I had walked into a lamp post.

I didn't like drinking or feeling out of control around Z, so my bulimia became progressively worse than it had been before. I would find myself standing in a supermarket queue with a basket of binge food, going in and out of the illness in my head. A well part of my brain told me to put the basket down and run, and yet the sick part kept telling me to go through with it. Z accused me of being a middle-class girl with a posh-girl disease when she found out about the bulimia during one of her drunken rants, which showed how little she knew about me and where I'd come from. I knew I was wasting my hard-earned money and damaging my body but I had an addiction to purging that wasn't dissimilar to her own experience with drugs and alcohol.

I didn't tell my mum what was going on. If I had, this period of my life might not have gone as badly as it did. I should have left sooner. But I was scared of Z and every time I tried to walk away she would turn up at my flat and shout outside my window. My neighbour called the police more than once, and sometimes the only way to escape was to leave through the back gate and get on a night bus until I felt safe enough to return home.

Z was known for her violence among the regular crowds we saw on nights out. We both got thrown out of a monthly queer night in a squat. It was a wholesome DIY spot in a former Chinese takeaway in Dalston, where people came to eat vegan food and step up to an open mic. Z started a fight while I was in the loo and we were told to leave. She pushed me to the floor when we were outside while people cradling mugs of herbal tea looked on, probably relieved they'd got rid of us. Z fell asleep on the bus home but started kicking me when we got off near her flat. I was worn out. I shoved her off, planning to leg it away from her, but I was stronger than I thought. She went crashing backwards through the window of a basement flat. I stood there blinking at the shattered glass, thinking *will I get arrested for this?* It was the only time I had fought back. I apologized to the residents, who were remarkably understanding, and called the police for them so they would have a crime reference number. Two officers turned up and as I was explaining that it was my fault and that I'd pay for the damage, a bag of weed fell out of my back pocket.

'Been smoking a bit tonight, have you?' the cop asked, eyebrows raised. I panicked and blurted out the truth: 'No, I only scored a few hours ago.'

'It's alright, you seem like a decent person.' He glanced over at Z, who was checking that the bottle of brandy in her coat pocket was still intact. 'Well done for letting us know about the window, we'll take it from here.' Maybe the police officer could tell I had enough on my plate that night or maybe he couldn't be bothered to deal with possession of a Class B drug. Either way, I've got myself out of some scrapes in my time, and that was unquestionably one of them.

I stayed with Z on and off for three years. I was still with her when she got clean through a lengthy heroin replacement programme. The day she came off Methadone was hard to watch. She had been taking 5ml of the green liquid medication for several months and the doctor agreed it was time to stop. She came to my place and slept. Then the sweats started, and she was vomiting and shitting, snot streaming down her face. I made a giant pot of daal. She'd eat and then be bent over the loo again. This continued for several days and then it was as if she had been reborn. I didn't recognize her. She was happier, CBT was working, and she was excited about looking for a job. But I realized I was still scared of the person she used to be and was waiting for the day she would lash out again. I finally left for good, and that time she didn't follow me.

I was twenty-five after the Z years, shell-shocked and direc- tionless. I was angry at myself for wasting all that time and for letting her hurt me. I needed to reinvent myself, to start again. One day I went out and had my hair chopped off. Thick chunks of my long down-to-my-bra-strap tresses fell to the salon floor and I was left staring at a short crop with an asymmetrical fringe. I wanted to be invisible again, sex-less, genderless, androgynous, and sexually unavailable. I was happy with what I saw. I looked like me or at least the me I wanted to get to know. Going for such a stylized look achieved the opposite of what I intended. It seemed to make me more visible – particularly to homophobic abuse: 'Urgh, is that a boy or a girl?' was regularly shouted after me on walks about town. It wasn't just my hair that changed. After a three-year hiatus off the mat, I went back to yoga to find myself. The poses didn't feel familiar anymore. I felt like a visitor to the practice, but I kept searching for that mystical thing I had tasted at the YMCA. If I kept looking I might find it again. Although I felt a lot of anxiety and alienation at that time and my relationship with my body was in a bad place, I started practising yoga daily again, racing to classes every night with different teachers. I was using the practice like a drug, as a way to keep my body moving and to stay away from thinking about eating and not eating, which was still an issue.

I Love the Smell of Newspapers in the Morning

In 2006, I decided to pursue my dream of being a news journalist. I had been writing for a long time and had done work experience at several newspapers and glossy mags before such as *Harper's Bazaar* and *Vogue*. I had started a blog and wrote reviews for websites by blagging freebies to gigs and LGBT club nights, which gave me access to a social life. I got short-listed for the Vogue Talent Contest for Young Writers in 2001, which boosted my confidence, but none of these moves had led to getting a job. I discovered that I needed the news industry's standard qualification to get a foot in the door so I enrolled on a full-time course in newspaper journalism at Harlow College in Essex. After that, things took off.

I landed my first paid writing job on a local newspaper in a Tory-run North London borough, where people complained about bins being collected only fortnightly and where more kids were starting to carry knives. I talked to gang members, NHS bosses, and government ministers at the start of their political careers (Boris Johnson was a regular visitor to the area when he was Mayor of London). I loved newspapers, the smell of them, what they stood for (telling the truth), the deadline-driven buzz of newsrooms and the inky-stained grubby-fingered business of being in places you shouldn't be. I discovered a passion for telling stories, campaigning about important issues and amplifying the voices of those that went unheard.

After two years I moved on to a paper in South London, and at the same time I met another older woman. She was an American graphic designer and DJ who was gentle, grounded and cool. She would make me music mixes on CDs and slip them into my backpack when I wasn't looking. I loved going to clubs, sitting behind decks and watching her orchestrate everyone's moves on the dance floor. Life was dreamy and fun at last. We moved in together and I started going to support groups for eating-disorder recovery when she told me she couldn't stand watching me hurt myself. I didn't want to lose her, so I made a commitment to get better. I wasn't ready to settle down but we had a civil partnership when her visa was due to run out so that she could stay. It was a beautiful day with me in a pretty dress, a ceremony in Hackney Town Hall with our closest friends and picnic with champagne in our local park. But I couldn't stick the relationship out. The recovery groups weren't working and my job was taking its toll. It was time to move on. I found a flatshare in South London to live closer to work and asked her to agree to dissolve the partnership the following year. I waited until her status to remain in the UK had been secured. It felt like the decent thing to do since I broke her heart. I was twenty-seven and this was only my second relationship. She loved me, even though I was hard to love at the time because I was still starving, binging and purging and had unpredictable mood swings. She was kind to me in all the ways I would now want a partner to be, but I didn't believe I deserved her love back then.

My news patch at the South London paper was Lambeth, where teenagers were being murdered regularly. Guns, gangs and knife crime were rife and it was almost always teenagers and young Black men who were dying. Several times a week I met families who were grieving the loss of their children to violence. I visited too many bereaved mothers during that time. I got used to it but it never got easier. I wrote a lot of front-page stories and started drinking a lot of red wine. It was an anaesthetic against the pain that surrounded me. Numbing myself was the only way to get through it. I kept drinking and vomiting, trapped in the same old cycle. The newspaper I was working at was known locally as the South London Depressed (mostly because we covered so much crime), which could also have been the theme for that phase of my life. The crime stories felt most important to me, but we had to cover local authority issues too, which meant going to dull council meetings. Drinking was the only way I had to switch off when getting home late after an evening in a draughty room listening to committees of mostly men discussing things that might never happen.

Although I was starting to drink far too much, yoga was still there too and in 2008 my practice took a different direction. Fed up with banging out energetic Ashtanga and Vinyasa classes without any joy, I needed something new. I found myself at a small studio that offered Mysore-style Ashtanga Self-practice, something that I had previously avoided because I thought you had to be spiritually advanced in order to practise in this way. This method follows the Ashtanga sequence but you practise alongside others in silence, alone but together. It has a more contemplative and meditative feel because it's so quiet. The teacher doesn't instruct but moves around the room like an angel offering assistance, guidance and – most importantly – love as you move through your practice. This was a pivotal year for me and the benchmark from which all my subsequent years of practice came. Gingi, my new teacher, owned the studio in Clapham, which was closer to my then home in Brixton. He was also the first teacher I felt a personal connection with, someone who I felt cared about his students. He would see me fighting with postures and gently encouraged me to stop doing that. He showed me how to practise in a way that was more compassionate and forgiving towards myself. I hadn't noticed I was being so hard on my body before I arrived at Gingi's place. I still resisted his suggestions sometimes and tried to force my body to do things it wasn't ready for, but I started to become aware of those urges for the first time. I was still turning up hungover and full of shame for drinking too much but I was happier with where yoga was taking me.

I would detox my emotions and go home to re-tox, but I also felt myself becoming part of a yoga community for the first time. Getting on my mat with the same people and teacher several times a week gave the practice a new meaning to me.

I realized that this was what I wanted – to belong somewhere. At long last, it felt like I was starting to own my practice. It felt like less of a burden and something I looked forward to. The yoga was mine to integrate and interpret, and it started becoming less of an exercise to keep myself moving or purge the abuses I was inflicting on my body and more about something deeper. It took me back to those early classes with my mum. At the Clapham studio I felt that we were all on different personal journeys but somehow travelling together when we breathed and moved in the company of each other. This feeling didn't stay with me when I left the studio, but it was present while I was there and that was enough. There was a juxtaposition emerging. I felt calm, contained and safe when I went to practise with Gingi, which was the opposite of how I felt about things in the rest of my life: depressing news writing, unstable emotions and alcohol abuse. It felt like yoga was the only thing sustaining me.

It was at one of those dreary council meetings that seemed to take for ever to end that I met a man and walked into a relationship without knowing what was going on. I went for a drink with him, thinking he might be a useful contact to dispatch juicy stories to me for the newspaper. But he had other plans. I was terrified the first time he inched closer to kiss me. I didn't know what to do and I didn't really want to do it but it wasn't long before we were an item. It didn't feel right at all because I preferred the company of women and was sure I was gay, but life would be easier if I tried to be straight so I went with it anyway. Big mistake.

My new boyfriend had a relatively visible profile in the community and refused to be seen with me in public for fear of being accused of leaking stories to the newspaper I worked for. This meant that we ignored each other at council meetings and had to arrive and leave the local cinema separately to avoid being spotted together. I can't believe I put up with it, but I was a first-timer when it came to having a relationship with a man and I wasn't sure how to do it.

It was a confusing time. The drinking, crime stories and a brief dalliance with antidepressants didn't mix well and that relationship hurtled to a crescendo when we were on holiday in Greece. We had been drinking single malt on a balcony at the villa and I didn't know my limits. Whisky knocked me sideways within minutes, changed my personality and rewired my brain. I started picking a fight and my boyfriend locked me in a tiny bedroom in an attempt to calm me down. I sat on the floor, back to the door, hugging my knees, feeling an eddy of anxiety and fury building in my chest. I was drunk. I was pissed off, embarrassed and tearful about the wreckage my life had become. My head was banging with thoughts:

Why am I drinking?
Why can't I stop?
Maybe it's a full moon.

I had to get out of there. I found myself unbolting the window, thinking *I'm overreacting, what's wrong with me?* I jumped out and ran to the nearby beach. It was as I was standing in the Mediterranean Sea that night that it first crossed my mind that alcohol might not be serving me. I didn't know who I was anymore. Drinking, which once soothed pain and thickened my skin to the grief I was writing about at the newspaper, wasn't working anymore. I wasn't meant to be a drinker anyway: although I wouldn't have described myself as a devout Muslim, it never felt right that I was the drunkest person I knew.

'Look at the moon!' I shouted, pointing at it when I saw

my boyfriend walking towards me, his face grey with terror. He waded in to pull me out and I tried to run away but he grabbed me. I felt relieved and held together for a moment as we stood in the water. Life would be calmer now. Except it wasn't. The next day, after we got back to London, he said it was over. I decided never to trust a man who thought wearing red trousers was a strong look ever again.

It was clear from that holiday that the burden of writing the stories of so many distraught parents each week was taking a toll on my mental health. I was still practising with Gingi, but alcohol was dominating my life and yoga couldn't compete. That night in Greece could have been a turning point but a few days after my relationship broke up I was sitting on the floor in my underwear in the basement flat where I lived, surrounded by bottles again. I cried into a keyboard, writing an email to my friend John, to tell him I didn't know how to stay alive anymore. It was my first call for help. John, a playwright who I knew would be awake in those early hours, was also decades sober. I needed someone like him to talk some sense to me. He wrote back immediately:

I love you. I love you in lots of ways. I love all the things you do, and I love the centre of you. I love the fact of waking up in the morning knowing you are alive, your existence warms the air. You know why you get addicted, why we all do, it's been eating, it's now booze, it's the same at the bottom of it, the way we think about ourselves, and how we can get through life. You are loveable, you are a fine, talented, clever, artistic, vulnerable, strong compendium of lots of sparkling things, and I love you because you are very easy to love. I would love you if you were hard to love, by the way.

My heart was starting to crack open at this point. I didn't believe John but what he said next snapped me out of my malaise.

> *On suicide, no – I had that as well, know what you are feeling. Why no? Because of other people really. I don't want to stand by your grave, however fantastic a film it would make, e.g. with Chopin's Funeral March and the vicar reading Psalm 22/23 'Yea though I walk through the valley of the shadow of death' in black and white, aspect ratio 1.33:1 like the '50s films. I would much rather be with you in real life, because you have no idea how crucially important you are to other people. Stop worrying about the booze, and the bulimia. They are significant battles to beat, but it's not a mountain, just a few small hills. You will stumble through.*

The next day, still feeling drunk, I called in sick at work then cycled to a local community alcohol and drug centre. I waited for four hours before they took blood tests, which found no alcohol in my system. The doctor said it looked like I metabolized it quickly and since I didn't drink all day, it was unlikely that I had a problem. The medic told me I was fine, just like the doctor had told my mum nothing was wrong when I didn't want to eat. Deep down I knew something was disturbing me, but whatever it was felt too unbearable to face. If an alcoholic needs permission to keep drinking, that message from the doctor at the rehab centre was definitely it for me.

I couldn't change my drinking so I switched my job. I left the South London paper and started working night shifts at a national newspaper. I stopped practising yoga because there was no time for classes. I just worked and drank and did little else for about a year. When you don't have to get up early and can't sleep at night, you've created the perfect conditions to keep drinking. My shifts were usually from 5 p.m. until 2 or 3 a.m. I'd get a taxi home where I'd drink a hidden bottle of wine (problems such as these must be concealed in wardrobes from flatmates). I'd get to sleep at 4ish, rise at 11 a.m. hungover, go to work and repeat the cycle. There was a gym in the building so I started running on a treadmill when I was given a break. I didn't enjoy it but it kept me busy and is probably what stopped me drinking on the job. At other times I'd lie a jumper on the floor in a disabled toilet no one used at that time of night and do a headstand to try to cure my permanent hangover. Or I'd sit on the floor and try to breathe slowly. I was clinging to these scraps of yoga from my former practice because I knew what to do even if it didn't always feel like it was working.

When I did the 1 a.m. to 9 a.m. shift, my mum would stay up late and keep me company. 'Nadi, are you okay?' she would ask, and I would usually start crying. 'Yeah, don't worry,' I'd tell her. 'Go to bed. You don't have to call me every day,' I'd tell her, sliding down my seat so the driver wouldn't see my teary face. 'Of course I worry about you. I want to call you, darling. You're my baby.' Which made me cry more. I was crying because I felt broken. I hated myself and hated that job. She would stay on the phone with me for the entire journey, talking in her soothing voice. 'I know this is hard. You won't have to do this for ever. Stay strong and remember that I love you so much, Jaan.' I didn't want those phone calls to end. I'd ring off and walk through the office doors sobbing because being reminded that someone loved me made me realize how little I loved myself.

* * *

John suggested I try one of the alcohol fellowships that had helped him. It was a comfort being with other people who know the disease that leads to powerless drinking. I met so many lovely people who were like me and had turned their lives around.

I loved the community aspect because I was craving somewhere to belong again. There's something remarkable that happens when you bring yourself to admit to another person that you've been so drunk you've pissed yourself, been sick on your bedclothes and fallen into bed with the wrong people and they say 'I've done that too'. There is freedom and a huge sense of relief in an honest admission. Even more remarkable is how I met so many people in those rooms who wanted to help me without expecting anything in return. It's called service – which it's said keeps you sober. I took on this service approach when I started teaching yoga. Of course I got paid, but the desire to help people was the biggest reason that kept me doing it. I spent several years going to meetings, managing a day sober and then relapsing. The recovery programme teaches you that you have to be willing to go to 'any lengths' to stay sober. At that time I wasn't. But now I look back and, though I found my own path to sobriety outside those meeting rooms in the end, I see their point. Any lengths, doing whatever it takes. There really is no other way.

I confessed to my mum in 2015. Telling her I had a drink problem was one of the hardest things I've ever had to do – even more than coming out as gay. I felt so much shame because of the faith she had tried to instil in me that forbade it. She has never had a drink in her life so I felt I was betraying her. But my mum couldn't have been more understanding. It made me wish I had told her sooner.

'I'm here to support you in any way you need,' she said,

'but you have got to do whatever it takes, Nadi.' It was the tough love I needed but perhaps not tough enough.

I promised her I would continue going to recovery meetings and get back to yoga. Committed to getting better, I walked out on the night shifts and started practising early-morning Ashtanga in the Mysore style again. The drinking didn't leave me, so it was hard getting out of bed at 5 a.m. to get to a studio and then to the office where I was now working at a newspaper during the day. But I practised as often as I could. I started to think I would never be able to stop drinking and reasoned that yoga might help me manage it somehow. I did finally stop drinking later that year, but not without crashing into a brick wall first. I didn't even want to stop drinking then, but I was on my knees, crying fat snotty tears in the toilet when my mum, heartbroken at this point, heard me. It was Christmas Day at my aunt's house in Oxford. I'd taken three bottles of wine from the kitchen and had been creeping upstairs to her bedroom to drink them throughout the day. I binged through a loaf of bread in the kitchen and made myself sick while the rest of my family chatted and played board games. Then I drank some more. No one seemed to notice I was getting louder, slurring my words, and not paying attention to anything anyone was saying. Nobody except my mum, that is. I had no idea how drunk I was until I ended up in the loo. 'Nadi, what's wrong? Let me in,' my mum demanded, tapping on the door.

'Go away,' I told her, knowing deep in my heart that she was the only person I trusted to help me. I heard her outside the door again a few minutes later and let her in. I didn't have to explain. 'We're leaving,' she said, and I knew this was it. There was no going back. My mum drove me to her home in London. I ran upstairs to my old bedroom and barged into a bookshelf that came crashing down. Mum shoved me into the shower. I stood under the water, wishing it could clean me on the inside. I knew my mum wasn't going to trust me to do this alone again and I was scared of the road that lay ahead.

The next day I woke up at 5.30 a.m., crawled over the books still on the floor and found half a bottle of red wine in my bag. I drank it and went downstairs to face my mum. I found her searching for rehab centres on an iPad. My life changed that morning. I refused residential rehab because I didn't want to leave my job or put a financial burden on my mum. But I did go to another community health centre. I turned up in an apologetic heap, saying 'I know I look okay and doctors don't think I've got a problem but I really have. PLEASECANYOUHELPME?' I'll always remember the woman on the front desk who became my alcohol support worker. Her name was Sapphire. She was at least a decade younger than me but had an aura of someone who had seen it all before. I don't know what I would have done if she had turned me away like the other rehab place had. Luckily she believed me and that's what saved me.

Staying sober was a nightmare at first. It was a worse hell than drinking had been. My mum called me every day to check how I was doing – I was a trembling wreck. I had been permanently numb when I was drinking and suddenly I was raw all over my body, like I had sunburn and was feeling absolutely everything. Lights were brighter, noises louder and other people were impossible to be around. I couldn't practise yoga anymore. Not Ashtanga anyway. My love for it meant that it didn't feel right when I hadn't respected the practice or taken it seriously. But I needed something. I started going to hot yoga classes, which I had never seen the point of so hadn't done before. The heat was intense and staying in the room felt impossible at first but I did thirty classes in thirty days in my usual all-or-nothing way. I kept going back to that studio for two years almost every day even when I was bored of it. Those classes were purely exercise and were nothing about building myself spiritually. The teachers also often sounded like they were reciting scripts as they instructed us into the postures. I wasn't inspired by that version of yoga but the classes worked in the way I needed at the time. The high temperatures calmed the anxiety I felt shaking inside me every day, and I would be lying if I didn't admit the heat was addictive. I replaced one addiction with another, but at least I didn't feel any shame about the new one.

In 2016, four months after that catastrophic Christmas Day, I relapsed on a work trip in Paris on my own in a hotel with three cans of supermarket beer. It wasn't a massive binge but it wasn't good. I had just started a part-time yoga teacher training course in London and knew I had to get back on the wagon quickly if I was to continue the course. I moved in with my mum and stayed with her for a year. I haven't had a drink since, which amazes me to this day because I spent so long thinking I wouldn't be able to live a life without alcohol. Now I can't imagine my life with it.

It's a miracle how we can change. People are sometimes shocked when I tell them I had a drinking problem because, apparently, I don't look like an alcoholic. But that's the biggest lie about this illness. Hardly any of us look like one and it doesn't discriminate. Who knows if I was an alcoholic or not? It doesn't matter what we call it. I was annoying, volatile, and embarrassing when I was drunk, I'd say those are enough reasons to stop. But there were many times I thought I wouldn't succeed because destructive behaviours like heavy drinking are driven by unidentifiable pain. Too many of us think we're beyond repair or that we don't deserve help when we're deep in our addictions. Neither is true. I love everything Gabor Maté says about addiction and he gets to the heart of it straight away in the introduction to his book *In the Realm of Hungry Ghosts*,[4] where he writes: 'All drugs – and all behaviours of addiction, substance-dependent or not, whether to gambling, sex, the internet or cocaine – either soothe pain directly or distract from it. Hence my mantra: The first question is not "why the addiction?" but "why the pain?"'

I thought I lacked the willpower to stop drinking but there's no will in the world that will heal a wounded heart. The only solution to the pain is working through the pain. I'm still working through it. Stepping into recovery is an ending but it's also the best beginning. Recovery doesn't have a fairytale ending. It's a slow, and in my case bumpy, road. It's raw and for me has meant hurting loved ones, and making amends often. There's no finish line. You just keep going, one day at a time, quickly, slowly, backwards, forwards. It's all worth it because learning how to live an honest life is what you gain.

When I was several months sober, still practising hot yoga and working as a communications manager in an office job and feeling on top of things for the first time in years, I met James. It was probably too soon to be getting involved with anyone. I hadn't found my groove with sobriety yet but I couldn't let him pass by. I was sure that I was ready for the next phase of my life. In fairness, so was he.

We were both thirty-six and I felt an urgent need to get life moving and find some joy, having squandered so many years in despair. James was gentle and kind, patient and forgiving – unlike every other man I had ever been with. He didn't scare me or want to change me. He was also interested in yoga and would drop everything to listen whenever I wanted to discuss the latest bit of philosophy I had on my mind or excitedly wanted to show him a posture that I had been practising and had managed to get myself into. When I met James I didn't feel straight or gay or anything anymore. It didn't matter because it felt right and I loved him. He represented safety and a compelling future I never thought I would find. I was bowled over and heady with hope. I pinned all my future dreams on our new union. I had to. I needed something to believe in and it became the two of us. If we stayed together for ever, life might turn out alright after all, I thought.

I Don't Know Where Hope Comes From

You know that thing when it feels as though your heart will break? Or that it won't burst when you really want it to because it already has? Your chest is filled with anger and sadness, tightness and no breath. You practise as best you can but just don't know if you're going to make it. You're scared.

Your friends tell you it will pass, and your mum promises it will get better. But it feels too brutal. You don't believe them. Even though you've been here before: when the only lover who mattered broke up with you, when friends disappointed you and your dearest died. You don't believe anyone. You meditate but the thoughts won't be still. You practise and nothing shifts. This goes on for months. The only thing keeping your bones together is knowing that it can't get worse than this.

Then one day you get out of bed. You slept terribly again, and everything still hurts. But you stare out of the window and LAUGH. At yourself, at this pain. You're laughing because there's nothing else to do. Your friends were right. Life went twisty, turny, topsy turvy and just plain rough. Nothing big has happened to change things; the events remain the same.

Yet here you are, willing to clamber to the surface again. You can still feel the darkness, but there is light peering in.

You've no idea how but could this be hope coming back? Whatever it is, you'd better grab it. You go for a walk, run, walk: fast drums and heavy bass pounding your ears as you move through the trees – WITHOUT A COAT, SILLY – so your legs, your fingers, your everything start to freeze. It seems as though autumn's here already. But you don't care, you wish it was raining, trusting nature to take care of you. You feel ALIVE, and you haven't felt that in a long time. Those bruises in your heart may still be there, and you know that it's entirely possible that you'll be doubled over in pain and tears again soon.

But you're starting to contemplate that sunnier times could lie ahead. Who knows if this will stick around, but for today – just for today – that'll do.

You know that feeling? That.

Dedicated to anyone who has felt like giving up for a little bit. Or still feels like they might want to (but not really because there's something inside you that really, really doesn't like giving up). There's no way around it but through it. This isn't easy and might mean that everything hurts for a while. It'll take as long as it takes. But turns out, it does get better. It always gets better.

CHAPTER 4

Who, What, Where, When Yoga?

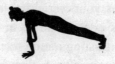

Now you know more about me, it's probably time to talk about the issue at hand: yoga itself. And lay all cards on the table to reveal what it actually is. Along with a bit more about what it definitely isn't. I might have been disillusioned with yoga by the time I met those teenage boys at the community centre, but it was because of the crazy journey I've had with the practice myself. I had spent so many turbulent years trying to get to grips with the spiritual aspects of yoga that when I became a yoga teacher I was confused. Spirituality seemed to be missing in the new classes I was seeing pop up as well as what was happening to yoga on social media.

The spiritual side to the practice isn't easy to condense because yoga is thousands of years old, vast and complex. Countless academics have written papers and books on yoga's meaning as well as its history with sometimes conflicting viewpoints. Some scholars claim yoga postures were influenced by Swedish gymnastics, others provide evidence that yoga came from ancient Egypt, while others such as the Hindu American Foundation launched their Take Back Yoga campaign in 2008 aimed at claiming the practice as Hindu in its roots. Many historians – unlike me – have dedicated their lives to the study of yoga and the sources of its traditions. I won't try to compete with them because I only have my own experience to go on. But I'll try to give you a sense of the philosophical side of the practice, which has helped me return to yoga all those times when it felt impossible to step on my mat.

In her book *Teaching Yoga, Adjusting Asana*,[5] Melanie Cooper, one of the tutors on a yoga teacher training course I did in 2016, sums up wonderfully the importance of understanding what yoga philosophy can mean for each of us personally. She writes: 'It [yoga philosophy] spans thousands of years and takes in a huge range of different viewpoints. Secondly, in order to teach something, you really need to understand it yourself and have a fairly clear idea of what you think and feel about the issues. It can often take years of study and thought to begin to know what you believe and what it means to live by your beliefs. Thirdly, spirituality can be a very sensitive topic for students. Some people may feel that yoga's spiritual aspects interfere with their own spiritual practice or that they challenge or imply disrespect to their beliefs. It is obviously important not to preach. Equally though, you would be leaving out a huge component of yoga if you were never to mention spirituality at all.'

Because her book is a manual, Melanie refers to the way yoga teachers might approach yoga spirituality in order to teach their students, but there's good guidance here for us all. Melanie makes important points in terms of how long a spiritual journey is likely to take and also how sensitive and personal it can be. I don't think the spiritual side of yoga should be forced on anyone because I believe it's best for people to find their own way. When I teach and meet people new to the practice, I always explain what it was intended for. I don't advocate throwing bucketloads of philosophy at people – I doubt I would have responded well to that as a beginner. That said, simple and regular acknowledgement is a good start. When new students aren't told about the wider framework of yoga, they don't know what they're missing out on. They might of course decide that it's not for them, but they should be given the big picture so that they have a choice. I also don't think it's wrong to come to yoga for the physical benefits alone – that's often the vehicle to get us started, as it was for me. Over time we might go deeper, as the practice and its radical potential opens up and reveals itself to us. It's not a process that should be forced or rushed.

I believe we're all spiritual beings at our core and we'll tap into that side of ourselves if and when we're ready. It took me long enough to do that and there will be others for whom it doesn't come easily either. We all practise yoga for different reasons: some enjoy the physical aspect, others might be looking for an emotional connection with themselves that brings with it an inner peace, and many others might want to go on a spiritual journey. Our desires and aims will vary, but what makes us stay with the practice is usually that it makes us feel better in some way and that's the only reason I think any of us need to get started.

History, unlike science, is told through different lenses depending on who is telling the story. It's open to interpretation and framing it in our own ways. So while I'll try to be as non-partisan as possible, what I'll be sharing here will inevitably be subjective and influenced by my own outlook and experience. This is the way I see things. I'm not an academic, historian or expert and none of it is intended to be presented as hard facts.

In terms of yoga's origins, I see it two ways: there are facts (as much as they can ever be) that history books will tell us, and then there is the truth, which is what I see as a person's own private relationship with yoga. A yoga practitioner's own experience, their questions and truth is also where the beating heart of yoga in practice is. This is a practice to be lived, not one that belongs in textbooks. I say this as someone who has learnt more about yoga through taking action rather than following a set of rules written in ancient texts. At the same time, it would be wrong to ignore the scriptures entirely for they contain valuable guidance and are fascinating – if confusing at times – in their wisdom. I think it's only possible to understand them more deeply on a personal level by questioning them and thinking about what they might mean in our modern lives.

A Brief History

The origins of historic Indian traditions are notoriously difficult to date. What we do know is that in ancient India, oral traditions were originally the main method through which religious and spiritual practices were passed down. I learnt about this on my degree course in the early noughties. It was enlightening to discover that the reliance on oral traditions was because there were no materials with which to write things down. It's believed that later, when ideas were documented, many texts deteriorated or were possibly eaten by insects. The texts that survived were later pieced together and many have formed books that continue to be studied by academics and Sanskrit scholars today.

In my research, I've found that yoga emerged sometime between 2,500 and 10,000 years ago so we don't have exact dates. Before yoga, the Indus Valley Civilization (2500–1500 BCE) is where the earliest traces of yoga were discovered, though they're vague and very different to what became modern yoga. The Vedic period (*veda* means knowledge) followed (1500–500 BCE) and spiritual practices around this time involved elaborate rituals to cultivate connections between the individual, the world and the heavens. Scriptures that have survived from this time were written in the ancient language of Sanskrit. The Vedas are sacred texts from this period, containing hymns, poems and mythological tales. There are four Vedas, filled with details of mystical rituals pertaining to a specific religious order. People at this time were preoccupied with finding connections between the realms of the body and the world. They did this through performing rituals and sacrifices during which they frequently consumed Soma – a plant-based juice believed to contain powerful spiritual properties, which might also have been hallucinogenic. It was believed that a greater knowledge of the different worldly realms granted one power over themselves. The idea was that if you controlled the body and understood the connection between the body and the outer world, you could then control the world.

The Upanishads are sacred texts that came later and were compiled between 700 and 500 BCE. It's been estimated that there are between 108 and 200, although there could be many more. These contain the beginnings of philosophy and mysticism in Indian religious history. Upanishad loosely translates as 'sit by or near', referring to the student sitting with their teacher to gain spiritual knowedge. Because the Upanishads constitute the concluding portions of the Vedas, they are referred to as Vedanta (the conclusion of the Vedas), and they serve as the foundational texts in theological discourses of many Hindu traditions. It's perhaps for this reason that yoga is often linked to Hinduism. It's believed that the *Bhagavad Gita* was written between 400 BCE and 200 CE. Like the Vedas and the Upanishads, the authors of the Gita are unclear but this Hindu scripture is also considered an important text in the context of practising yoga. Despite this, and because yoga comes with a philosophy rather than an allegiance to any deities, I've always seen it as a secular practice in my own life. Given that there was so much else culturally going on in India when yoga emerged, I've often been unsure about whether yoga has been co-opted by Hinduism as opposed to being a Hindu practice itself. I'm not saying these things are true either way but it's a big question I have without a definitive answer. I understand that Hinduism must interrelate with yoga in some capacity because of texts such as the Vedas, Upanishads and *Bhagavad Gita*, but it's confusing because not everyone agrees. It's a debate that's unlikely to ever come to an end.

There are people I've spoken to who support my views and there are others I know who are offended by this idea and maintain that denying yoga its Hindu roots is like rewriting history. It's not my intention to divorce yoga from Hinduism entirely, but I think – given yoga's vast and ancient origins that pre-date all religions that came later – there has to be more to it.

The Upanishads contain the first specific descriptions of yoga, mentioning practices involving control of the senses, and using the breath. To put this in context, this was also the era when the Buddha died (483 BCE) and Greek philosophers Socrates (born around 470 BCE) and Plato (born around 428 BCE) were also active, far away in the Mediterranean. Interestingly, in Buddhism, the term *anattā* refers to the doctrine of non-self, a belief that there is no unchanging, permanent self, soul or essence in living beings. This is the opposite of what is believed in yogic philosophy, where the aim is to connect with the Self or *atman* (soul) and realize its connection with a Supreme Self or being that will lead to an ultimate enlightened state.

So yoga existed during the Upanishadic and Vedic eras as a term for joining two things. The word yoga itself has several meanings. It's usually defined as the union of the individual consciousness with that of Universal consciousness (which could be interpreted as God, if we understand this as the ultimate supreme omniscient being of all). The word *yog* comes from the root word *yuj*, meaning 'to yoke' or 'to join', which is why yoga is so commonly associated with the idea of unifying the mind, body and spirit. I noticed very quickly that spiritual pundits (a Hindi term of respect for a wise person) I met when travelling on early trips to India, specifically in the north, often referred to yoga as simply yog. The A in yoga appears to be an English transliteration of the original term. In practice, specifically when we step onto our yoga mats, I think of the bridge that unites the mind and body as the breath.

In his book, *One Simple Thing*,[6] Eddie Stern says the ancient Sanskrit grammarian Panini wrote that there were two ways of defining the word yoga, depending on its usage. The first is *yujir*, which describes the action of joining – for example an ox to a cart. For yoga practice, which was classified as a spiritual discipline years later during the Upanishadic age, the correct derivation is from *yuj samadhan*, which means that yoga is a special kind of concentration called Samadhi: absorption. Our minds are naturally inclined towards absorption, whether in books, ideas, people, goals. The idea is that when we focus our minds on spiritual pursuits we can approach Samadhi – the deepest level of concentration, where we may gain knowledge of our inner selves. Though yoga has many meanings, future definitions of the practice still draw on this concept of joining two things in terms of connecting the essence of an individual's Self or atman with a transcendent reality.

After the Upanishads came the Yoga Sutras, which are believed to have been written sometime between 300 BCE and 200 CE. If you want to read more about the philosophy attached to yoga, then this is a good place to start. They are what I return to the most for their simplicity and I find them easier to understand than many of the other yogic texts. The translations I have found most helpful are *Yoga Sutras of Patanjali*[7] by Edwin Bryant and B.K.S. Iyengar's *Light on Yoga*,[8] which is perhaps the most widely read. The Sutras are usually compulsory texts on yoga teacher training courses. They can be read in a single sitting, though discussions on their meaning can go on for hours and even days or substantially longer. In my experience, one's understanding of the Sutras changes and deepens over time.

The Yoga Sutras

The sage Patanjali is credited with having written the Yoga Sutras, though not a lot is known about him (it's assumed Patanjali was a 'he'). Some practitioners believe Patanjali (or the many Patanjalis) lived around the second century BCE and also wrote works on Ayurveda (the ancient Indian system of medicine) and Sanskrit grammar. The Yoga Sutras form a guidebook filled with words of wisdom for how to live well, both for yourself and your community as a whole. There's a religio-spiritual element to them, which is no surprise given the Vedic and Upanishadic practices that preceded them. They form the philosophical framework that's attached to the physical yoga practice. The word *sutra*, which usually refers to an aphorism, means 'string' or 'thread': a beautiful metaphor for conveying how integral the physical and philosophical are to each other. In Ashtanga there is a series of movements performed between poses called vinyasas. I like to think of these vinyasas as a thread that links everything together, like prayer beads on a Mala commonly used in Hinduism, Jainism, Sikhism and Buddhism.

Without studying these important threads that form the Sutras, we're not really practising yoga within its wider context. The Sutras are four short chapters of 196 one-line verses that present what the goal of yoga is. They discuss: the difference between the mind and consciousness; enlightenment and its stages; the Eight-limb practices of yoga (more on this below; see page 82), and the powers of meditation.

Some of the Sutras are more complex than others. Many of them can be understood as simply as they are presented. Crucially, and this really is quite remarkable, only four of the Sutras mention Asana, the word that refers to the poses. This suggests that yoga postures didn't emerge straight away – the philosophy came first. One of my favourites is the frequently quoted Sutra 2.4: *sthira sukham asanam* (posture should be steady and comfortable), and it is fairly straightforward. I don't think this Sutra means that the poses are meant to be easy. Because of course they're not – they're rarely comfortable either. Many postures feel unnatural, because they demand that we do them in a way that is very different to the way we habitually move. Some of the poses are likely to feel uncomfortable when they are new – like I found doing that wonky Triangle Pose (Trikonasana) in the YMCA my first time. There's nothing natural about this pose. The energy is moving in different directions at the same time. Your feet are rooting down and pointing one way. The hips are squaring back, as the upper body moves sideways with one arm moving down, the other reaching up to the sky. Back bends are the same. They're excellent to practise for creating space in the tightest parts of our backs, but also unnatural in that we're turning our ribcage outwards, shoulders backwards and opening our hearts by reversing what our forward-folding spines do most of the time.

My interpretation of Sutra 2.4 is to observe and see if it's possible to breathe through the discomfort that might be present when doing certain postures. Discomfort is different to pain. It's important to stop if anything we're doing hurts. When I'm teaching, I encourage yoga students to go to an edge when holding postures where they feel sensation. I push them gently if it looks like they're having an easy time. This might mean it's hard to stay in the pose or takes intense concentration and effort to stay with it once there. I think that's important because there doesn't seem any point in practice if we're not challenging ourselves to explore. That's what makes the edge an interesting place to be. It's often through discomfort that we make discoveries and experience transformation.

At the same time, the practice isn't meant to be an endurance test so it's essential to recognize the difference between discomfort and pain. Discomfort is usually a feeling that might not feel pleasant at first but, if we stick with it, eventually something (physically, emotionally or both) will shift. I think it's part of the practice to learn to deal with discomfort and to breathe through it, much like we might when facing challenging times in other areas of our lives. In recent years, staying with discomfort on my mat, observing it, and almost holding it tenderly in my body rather than wishing it would go away has been about exactly that. Almost preparing myself to better deal with tough stuff that might lay ahead. This is something that needs practice regularly for me because for a long time I was very bad at doing it. The avoidance of pain was why I spent so long in the throes of binge drinking and bulimia and, though I have more practice now, I still find it hard to do.

Another lesser-quoted favourite of mine is Sutra 2.33, which has a whiff of CBT about it. It loosely translates as: 'When negative thoughts present themselves, cultivate and think the opposite thoughts'. Granted I didn't follow this advice much in my early yoga journey, and I don't think we can heal ourselves with positive thinking alone, but I like it because it makes sense. It often comes to my mind these days – usually quite late in the day – when I've been stuck in the middle of a difficult period in my life and suddenly realize part of the reason why I've let the pain drag on for so long is that I've forgotten to look for places I might find a glimmer of joy.

The Eight Limbs of Yoga: a Prescription for Moral Conduct and Self-discipline

In the Sutras, Patanjali mentions the Eight Limbs, which set out how yoga should be practised with a view to reaching enlightenment. The Eight Limbs are less commandments than guidelines for how to live a meaningful life with purpose. They demonstrate how to acknowledge the spiritual parts of our nature. I think about these a lot – particularly the first two, the Yamas and Niyamas, some of which are relatively easy to do – most of the time. *Ash* means 'eight' and *tanga* translates as 'limbs'. Ashtanga was designed to formally integrate and help practitioners approach these Eight Limbs in an organized and chronological way, but it's possible to observe the steps regardless of the style of yoga class you're practising and to do so in a different order. Postures are the gateway for many of us new to the practice, after all, although meditation and breathwork could be too.

The eight steps themselves offer practical ways in which to explore and discover the many wisdoms offered in the Sutras. They're meant to be a non-negotiable part of the practice of yoga but I sometimes look at the list of Yamas and Niyamas and think I'm not doing very well at them at all. Of course I slip up, but after I stopped drinking, when honesty became an important part of my recovery, I made a commitment to make better use of the Eight Limbs. Some of them mean more to me than others but I find them all a good benchmark to refer to. They form a moral compass or North Star.

Let's take a closer look at these Eight Limbs, and the tenets within them. I should add that these are only my latest interpretations; I interrogate them all the time.

1. Yama

There are five guidelines to strive for that set out an ideal way to live in order to be in harmony with ourselves and others.

Ahimsa: Non-violence

Ahimsa is about practising non-violence in our thoughts, intentions and behaviours. For many, this extends to following a vegan or vegetarian diet. It also means we should be committed to, and actively working towards a goal of equality and equity for all. It's about treating ourselves with kindness and not engaging in negative internal dialogue or self-sabotaging behaviour (not easy, right?). In our yoga Asana (posture) practice, it could be interpreted as not ignoring pain and forcing ourselves into postures our bodies aren't ready for, as well as not judging ourselves (or others) negatively (both on and off the mat).

Incidentally this is also usually the first tenet of yoga that trolls wheel out when they come after me on social media, alleging that something I've written has been violent in some way when all I was trying to do was tell the truth. I wonder what they'd make of this book.

Satya: Truthfulness

I like to think I'm relatively good at this one these days. After years of lying and living with shameful secrets, I finally value honesty. The first part of telling the truth of course has to start with ourselves. I think it's so important because if we can't be honest with ourselves what else have we got? I was lost for so many years because I couldn't be honest with myself. Satya refers to both words and thoughts, and not engaging in deceitful or misleading behaviour. Satya could also mean not using the truth unkindly or in a way that harms others (this is a useful one to remember when a loved one has disappointed you – I've failed many times at that). Ahimsa comes before Satya, so my understanding is that speaking or living in a way that we believe to be truthful shouldn't cause harm or violence.

Asteya: Not stealing

Aside from the obvious issue of taking what's not ours, this includes not thinking about stealing, and not taking more than a fair share of what's owed to us. I often think of this in terms of not stealing other people's time or asking too much from others and being fair and respectful of the energy and capacity they might have for what I'm asking them to do, which is also about being compassionate. I hate being late and keeping people waiting for me. When I am late, I become fixated on making sure I'm punctual the next time. I also always meet deadlines, though this takes less work because it's ingrained in me from my newspaper days. As a yoga teacher I think it's important I finish classes on time, and on the rare occasions I've run over I've let everyone know so that they have the choice to leave. I'm not a beacon of perfection at Asteya. This tenet could also be interpreted as not being wasteful or consuming to excess, and I've definitely failed at this in a big way with food and alcohol so it's very close to my heart to uphold this rule as best I can as a way to repent for the past.

Brahmacharya: The right use of energy

Brahmacharya is often linked to sex but it can also mean conserving our energy (creative, sensual and sexual) so that it's not leaking out in places that aren't useful to ourselves or others. Spreading ourselves too thin, burning all cylinders, or doing too much in other words. I sometimes fall into the trap of cramming in more than I can probably get done, or more than I have energy for and then can be left feeling drained, which then might mean I can't be present for others. In terms of sex, for monks and nuns this means abstinence and conserving sexual energy for spiritual purposes. For the rest of us, it might mean monogamy, being faithful, respectful and not behaving recklessly or engaging in sexual acts that might harm ourselves or others. I've not cheated in any of my relationships so thought I'd nailed this one. Then I started psychoanalytic therapy and found out just how complex sex can be and has been for me. My sexuality has never been straightforward for a start. The older I've got, the more I see sex for the powerful thing it is. Not just for me but for everyone I've been in significant relationships with. Sex is great and I think we're all more like animals than we might like to think. At the same time, we're not because we have more complex emotional intelligence than our fellow mammals, and with this comes a bigger responsibility. I think the idea with this Yama is that sex isn't just sex and if we believe it is, it'll catch up with us at some point and we'll have to look at our actions and deal with the consequences if we want to live functional and healthier lives. Complicated, isn't it?

Aparigraha: Non-greed

We might feel a sense of lacking something or that we're not good enough. This in turn can create feelings of attachment to belongings, relationships or status, and the fear of losing material things, which can make us unhappy. I tend to let material things go if I lose them. I also hate shopping so am not bothered about buying the latest thing on trend. Relationships are another matter. I fall in love very easily, am fiercely loyal and have willingly given my heart away too quickly to people who've then hurt me. In my experience attachments in relationships are very difficult to avoid because people in my life are important to me. I just don't know if it's possible to be measured in my attachments so that when they break down I won't feel pain. But I see the value in building a strong sense of self so that we're not greedy for approval and love, although that too can be hard to do. As is dealing with bereavement and grief.

2. Niyamas

These are four positive habits that relate to our treatment of ourselves.

Saucha: Cleanliness

This refers to cleanliness of the body, mind and environment. It could also refer to diet and abstaining from negative or unclean thoughts such as anger, greed, jealousy and unclean words. Swearing probably comes into this category and I'm afraid I'm never going to be good at cleaning that up, though Saucha probably refers to the intention behind our swearing. For example, swearing at someone in a fit of anger (not something I've done much at all in my life, it just doesn't feel right) will have a different effect to using a swear word when joking around. This Niyama makes me think of something a Parsi friend taught me: *Humata, Huxta, Huvarshta* (Good Thoughts, Good Words, Good Deeds), which is considered the core maxim of Zoroastrianism. Though not yoga, I love this as a simple set of actions to aspire to and it fits well with yoga philosophy.

Santosha: Contentment

This is slightly different to happiness, because it's based on an internal knowledge of ourselves rather than external circumstances. It feels to me to be about acceptance, which I sometimes think is the hardest thing to find in the world. Even harder than being honest, which comes more naturally to me than it did in the past. The key to true contentment is living in the present and being satisfied with where we are, rather than looking to external objects or people to make us happy. This is another one I struggle with because my emotions have been unstable for as long as I can remember. I pretend I'm thick-skinned when life gets tough yet, in reality, I'm incredibly porous and sensitive to things people say and do in relation to me. Living in this way isn't going to get me closer to Santosha so it's a big work in progress for me.

Tapas: Austerity/Transformation

This is one of my favourites because I'm a big believer in the power of transformation now that I've seen it happen in my own life, specifically with my changed behaviour around food and alcohol. Tapas means to overcome adversity and not give up when practice (or life) gets tough. The word itself comes from the root *tap*, which means 'to heat'. The heat generated from the physical practice of Ashtanga, for example, tends to make us sweat and this helps burn away impurities – physical, mental and emotional so it supports the earlier Yama of Saucha. The body becomes lighter and more flexible over time. I often think of this when postures are hard to do or life is difficult, or those excuses not to step onto my mat creep in. This reminds me of the power to be found in discipline. Life's hard, I tell myself, and I will get through, things will get better and hope will return – if I keep going, which means showing up for practice.

Svadhyaya: Self-study

This is about looking inwards, the study of ourselves, our thought patterns and reactions, and observing the things that prevent us achieving stillness of mind. Some of the ways I do this are by reading books, but mostly I do it through therapy and conversations with people closest to me who are doing the same. Community and being with others committed not so much to self-development for improved performance or productivity but to self-knowledge for the sake of understanding the human experience is important to me. In the context of my recovery, this Niyama might also mean knowing when it would be good to ask for help. If you're anything like me, life can start becoming a bit too unbearably solemn when searching for meaning and purpose all the time. So I think it's sometimes useful to let feelings ebb and pass through without having to work out what they mean. One of my biggest downfalls in the recovery fellowships was when mentors in the groups would tell me to 'hand it over', meaning let the gods/universe/

higher powers take care of it, and I was too busy trying to work out what that meant so couldn't. I also felt that the only way I was going to change was by doing it myself.

Trusting in a higher power or divine being felt too hard, felt like I was giving up control of my life in a way even when I could see how effective 'handing it over' seemed to be for other people. I see things differently now. There can be a lot of value in not intellectualizing everything and in trusting that the answers will reveal themselves to us in time.

3. Asana: Seat/Posture

At last, the limb that refers to the poses. Through the practice of Asana, we develop the habit of discipline and the ability to concentrate, both of which are necessary for meditation. Indeed, their aim is to prepare the body for meditation, which comes at the end of all yoga practice once the body has been loosened up and purged. This is why Savasana, Corpse Pose (the final, lying-down posture) comes right at the end. Imagine how busy the mind would be if we tried to do it at the beginning! Although some teachers bookend their classes with this pose, I sometimes start classes with a modified version with feet flat on the floor and knees pointing to the ceiling so that the posture is still a little active. Teaching a pose like this at the start of class can be a good way to set the tone of tuning into a meditative state before ending in the same posture to rest. Doing this can be revealing in terms of observing the state of the mind at the start compared with how it might be at the end of the practice. It's also a great way to notice any shifts that have taken place, which is something I always encourage students to do. Making a note of those shifts is often what keeps us coming back to practice.

I try to approach as many postures as I can in a meditative way when I practise so that when it comes to resting I'm best prepared. It's not always easy. Sometimes I find I'm racing through them, apparently in a rush to get to the end. Or I'm thinking about work that's piling up or emails that need a reply, which of course defeats the purpose. It's another work in progress. I take solace in the fact that the Sutras recognize the restless mind, which reminds me why I'm doing it. Yoga Sutra 1.2: yoga is the stilling of the changing states of the mind.

4. Pranayama: Breath Control

These are techniques designed to help us be in control of our own respiratory process, while recognizing a connection between the breath, mind and emotions in the body. There are so many breathing exercises in the yogic system and each has a specific purpose to align the body and mind. But not all Pranayama exercises are for everyone because breathing techniques can trigger anxiety or bring up difficult emotions in some people. I didn't enjoy any form of Pranayama when I first started practising yoga – particularly not the ones that involve breath retention. Holding my breath made me feel light-headed and anxious. I still approach techniques new to me with caution and always let students I'm teaching know that they can stop at any time if it doesn't feel right. Many of these practices can take a while to get used to. Nadi Shodhana (alternate-nostril breathing) is a classic. It's relatively easy to get the hang of and excellent for bringing a sense of balance within the body. That said, it took me a long while before I felt comfortable doing it regularly. I share a simple version of it as much as I can when teaching but always advise students to go gently. I once taught a class where a young woman said breathing exercises made her feel panicky but that she was keen to learn. I told her to take it slowly because these practices can be transformative so going slow (not just for her but for all of us) is a good approach. It's important to check in regularly and to stop when you've had enough. We don't have to stick these practices out to benefit or learn from them. It's far better to do little and often to help the body and mind acclimatize rather than dive in expecting life-changing results in an instant. There are still some Pranayama exercises that I avoid because I don't like how they make me feel. I might be missing out but I think that's okay because I tell myself I want a practice that cultivates compassion within myself. Or could it be that I'm delusional and avoiding discomfort that could potentially lead to transformation? It's a mystery.

5. Pratyahara: Sense Withdrawal

This stage is about making a conscious effort to draw our awareness away from the external world and stimuli. You can do this while practising Pranayama with your eyes closed, or to a degree when practising Asana by sending the Drishti (gaze) to a specific place. Ashtanga yoga, for example, specifies gaze points when practising Asana, such as looking at the big toe or a raised hand, to assist this process, but you can of course employ this idea in whatever style of yoga or postural practice you enjoy. I also think you can practise Pratyahara anywhere you might be: on public transport, on a busy station platform, in a crowded room as I often do simply by lowering my gaze, tuning in for a few quiet moments and becoming aware of my breath. Practising Pratyahara is an opportunity to step back, focus the mind and send the gaze inward.

6. Dharana: Concentration

Pratyahara creates the setting for Dharana. Once you've shut out the outside world, you can properly look at what's going on inside your head. This is tough when it's busy inside there. Often there's so much noise it's hard to make sense, which makes me feel as if I'd rather be doing something else. However, I remind myself that it's useful to look. My thoughts never form a coherent narrative and I have a capacity for containing a lot of them at the same time. People often tell me that I speak fast. I think this must be down to the speed of my thoughts, which can lead to a stream of consciousness in my speech (and writing) as my mouth (and fingers) clamber to keep up. Sometimes the thoughts fly past in a blur, at other times they're clearer even if disjointed or I don't like what they're telling me. This is why although I've never been diagnosed with Attention deficit hyperactivity disorder, I've sometimes wondered if I have traits.

It can feel impossible to switch the mind off, but you don't have to. Just watching the thoughts come and go rather than feeling an urgent need to act on them (very common, in my experience) is enough. Dharana has taught me a lot about patience and how the act of concentrating itself can slow the thinking processes down.

7. Dhyana: Meditation/Contemplation

Although Dharana and Dhyana might look very similar, there is a distinction between them. Concentration is about putting your focus on the mind and watching it, whereas this next stage is about being aware of the mind but without a fixed focal point. It's a fine line. Steps 6 and 7 might go hand in hand for a lot of us for a long time. It can take hours, months or even years to come to a place where the mind is familiar with how to quieten down. You've arrived at step 7 once you notice that the mind is quieter and produces very few thoughts – or, in some lucky people, there might no longer be any thoughts at all. It takes strength and stamina to get to this state. But it doesn't have to turn into a competition with yourself. My approach always boils down to practising and seeing what happens.

8. Samadhi: Ecstasy/Enlightenment

This final stage is referred to as the point at which the meditator transcends the Self. Through the practice of yoga, we're looking for a form of transcendence and the biggest mystery is that you don't know when it will arrive. Transcendence is the motivation for practice and our ultimate goal. The aim is to realize a deep connection to either the Divine, a Supreme Being or a sense of interconnectedness with all living things. Like the early civilians during the Vedic and Upanishadic periods. Samadhi is described as a sense of peace, liberation and a sense of oneness with the universe.

I realize it might seem a lofty goal. In the past I often questioned whether Samadhi might even be a lie. Could it be that we're all chasing this thing that might not exist? But how could I possibly know? And what happens when we get there? Does it mean we stop practising? Or does the cycle of practice just start again? Again, I don't know. The magical thing about Samadhi is that you can't buy it – just as you can't buy any of the positive benefits of these Eight Limbs. They have to be practised and integrated. Samadhi is also not something you can possess, meaning it's unlikely to be a permanent state. I like to think that it might be possible to experience glimpses into Samadhi in much the same way as the late Buddhist monk Thích Nhất Hạnh said that we can experience Nirvana – as a fleeting thing. Both Samadhi and Nirvana are goals we should aim for, and the only way to get there is to continue practising.

* * *

Before we go on, a note about Sanskrit: whose language is it anyway? Given its connection to ancient sacred texts, Sanskrit could be considered the language of the gods. But the world's oldest language can be a divisive issue. It's now largely obsolete and spoken by less than 1 per cent of Indians,[9] although there have been attempts made by modern Indian politicians to bring about its revival by reinstating it within the school education system. There are different groups who are for or against this because the language is closely linked with Hinduism.[10] It is being opposed most strongly by politicians from the southern state of Tamil Nadu (Tamil is not derived from Sanskrit) who believe India should be a secular state.[11]

Sanskrit originally belonged to an Indo-Aryan group of people who went to South Asia from Central Asia and Europe. It is the root of many (those that use the Devanagari script) but not all languages from the region. Urdu, for example, which is my mother tongue, uses the modern Persian script, which is itself a derivative of Arabic. Urdu, Farsi and Arabic, unlike Devanagari, are read from right to left. When it comes to Sanskrit and yoga, my take on it is that it's important to know the history of the language and be aware of how it fits within the history of South Asian civilization. I know the

Sanskrit names for poses I practise and teach but I use a mixture of both Sanskrit and English when teaching because it's more inclusive and I'm always teaching English speakers. I want people to understand and remember what I'm sharing. Teaching isn't about alienating, confusing or, it should be said, showing off. That said, I like to know what the postures mean in Sanskrit (because the translations aren't always on point) which gives a glimpse into history and old cultures. At the same time, it's not lost on me that another reason that Sanskrit can be controversial is because it was originally restricted for use only by people born into certain upper castes. It was banned to the lower castes or working classes,[12] which I assume was a way of denying them the knowledge found in the ancient texts. Doesn't sound so great now, does it? So, while I think it's good to have some insight into Sanskrit sounds and words (especially if you like chanting), it's worth being aware of its associations. I'm not massively fussed about chanting in Sanskrit, as lovely as it can be to listen to. Some of the sounds are hard to produce even for me as a bilingual South Asian person because, as I mentioned, my native language is Urdu. That said, I generally notice that South Asian yoga practitioners tend to find Sanskrit easier to get the hang of pronouncing correctly than others simply because we have access to some similar sounds in our languages and know how to use our tongue in the required ways, which English-only speakers don't. I tend to stick to the Ashtanga chants that appear at the beginning and end of the practice because I know them well and understand their meaning (as much as anyone can). So where does this leave you? I think learning about Sanskrit is good (particularly if you're a white yoga teacher or you'll end up looking like you don't care about the bigger picture of the practice). But in terms of using Sanskrit regularly, I can't say I do. I see its value, but it's fair to say I'm conflicted about it.

Black History and Egyptian Yoga

Like a lot of people, I've gone through twenty-five years of practice thinking of yoga as South Asian in origin. That's what many books tell us. But I stumbled across Smai Tawi online and was curious to learn more. Smai Tawi refers to a spiritual system of self-development created by the sages of Ancient Egypt. It's a healing and regenerative form of spirituality, characterized by a series of body postures combined with controlled breathing and meditation. It also comes with its own philosophy.

Some researchers say this practice could have pre-dated the traditions that emerged in South Asia and I wanted to know more. I started reading more about it and was fascinated by this history that seemed to be buried. I discovered that Kemetic Yoga was developed by studying, translating and interpreting hieroglyphic texts of Kemet (Ancient Egypt) and illustrations on the walls of temples. Like South Asian yoga, Smai Tawi is a spiritual system that is about practising to reach enlightenment. There appeared to be a big crossover, where both the Asian and African practices seemed to have the same goal. It made sense to me that similar practices designed to make sense of the natural cosmic order of life were going on in different parts of the world at similar points in history.

One question that confused me regarding the Egyptian practices was that they were called yoga, because yoga is a Sanskrit word. I made a phone call to my friend Amani Eke, who I knew would shed some light. I met Amani in 2017 at a retreat in Kent for women of colour where she was teaching Smai Tawi, and we became friends. I loved the classes she taught. The practice was slower and more methodical than what I was used to, but it also felt familiar breathing and moving in a specific way. We did a Sun Salutation in the Kemetic way and, although some of the postures that followed had different names that I didn't know, they were not entirely unfamiliar as I moved my body into them.

Amani explained the system to me:

The term Smai Tawi was used to describe the unity of Upper Egypt and Lower Egypt under one ruler. So Smai Tawi relates to us bringing union to the duality that lies within us all, our lower and higher natures, allowing us to find divine balance, which is known as Maat. Smai is also symbolic of the breath which contains a life force energy called Sekhem or Prana in the Indian system through the union or control of the lungs.

The practice of the physical postures was known as the Thef Neteru or Sema Paut, just like you have Asana in Indian yoga. It is important to understand the mythological teachings of each God and Goddess (Neter). The Neteru are really symbols of cosmic forces in nature and in the mind. Understanding their energies and the roles they play in each myth helps us to regain our power and awaken the cosmic forces which lie within our own consciousness.

Amani started exploring Smai Tawi in 2008 after discovering it through her study of ancient African history. She told me that when she started teaching, some people who attended her classes argued with her, claiming that yoga is Indian and disputing that it had any African links. Did she think it was the use of the word yoga in relation to these Egyptian practices that was causing the confusion or winding people up? She replied:

Smai Tawi is one of the original names for the practice, because obviously yoga is a Sanskrit word. When we talk about Kemetic Yoga we are really just using the word 'yoga' to market it because people understand that word. The symbol for Smai also has the meaning of union just like Indian yoga does. As much as you and I don't like it, the practice has been commercialized. At the same time, is it really a bad thing? At least it is a way of bringing these ancient practices to the masses.

I completely agree with Amani, but my problem has never been that yoga is now as popular as it is. I take issue with it being repackaged into something that it's not, of it being divorced from its roots, perhaps like the history of Smai Tawi has been buried. I asked Amani to tell me more about that.

There's a lot of Black history that is missing, not taught or has been hidden, which is down to ignorance really. Just because people haven't discovered or learnt about something doesn't mean it hasn't happened. What many people don't know is that there was a big link between North-east Africa and Asia. There are so many links between the two continents. That whole part of history is missing, or not talked about, but you can find it if you look for it. I think some people don't want to accept that Black people or any darker-skinned people of the earth had any input in history, science, astrology or maths.

In the UK, schools only teach post-slavery Black history, like we started as slaves, when we had many large civilizations that were in existence and thriving before many European ones. Most Europeans still refuse to accept Ancient Egyptians as being Black Africans. We are very vast in our features and colour, and actually when you translate terms and symbols you find out where the people are originally from.

Ancient Egypt was far larger than what it is today and modern-day Egypt was actually Lower Egypt not Upper. This is a known fact. People do not want to put two and two together because they will start to unveil many truths they are not ready to accept. But this is due to the media and so-called documentaries they listen to. Yet I'm sure they have never heard about any of these things I am talking about.

In terms of whether we're talking about Indian yoga or African yoga – and I've studied both – I feel they're the same. They're practised in slightly different ways. When you study Egyptian yoga you have similar principles to follow, the same as in Indian yoga philosophy. We also follow similar practices to the Yamas and Niyamas too. Things like breathwork, words of power or chants, meditation, self-observation, psycho-physical/ spiritual exercises, virtuous living, dietary purification, studying and practising wisdom teachings. They are both systems that help bring you closer to self-knowledge and reconnect with the original source. There are a few additional principles and guidelines to follow within Smai Tawi, but overall they're the same. I don't think of them as being very different. When I think of the word yoga I am thinking of my personal practice; it's about how I'm trying to align with myself and the Divine. It's about me striving for that enlightenment and trying not to be selfish or egotistical. We're practising for the same goal so there's no real difference.

I found speaking to Amani fascinating, to discover that practices with such similar principles at their core were going on in different parts of the world. Learning about Smai Tawi proved to me that it's important to keep an open mind when it comes to yoga, and how all of us, including me, have things to learn about the history of yoga practice. Speaking to Amani also made me think that ultimately whether yoga is exclusively Indian, or Egyptian or Hindu, doesn't really matter. I strongly believe it's important to acknowledge and respect all possible origins for yoga because colonialism never ends well, but when I come across arguments about 'taking yoga back' it makes me feel sad. I understand this backlash is against some of the problems I've talked about with the commodification of yoga in the West, but I still think there has to be a better way to reclaim these practices in a manner that's less about 'taking' and more about 'giving' them to more people. Like Amani says, we're practising for the same goal, so it feels like focusing on the similarities between practices rather than the differences and trying not to get bogged down with who yoga belongs to is the best way forward. Given how personal yoga is, like any other faith or spiritual practice, surely it belongs to us all.

Practise Each Pose as a Prayer

6 a.m., Friday morning

I wake up, groggy, grunty, not ready. But today is the day I go to practise with one of my teachers. Some mornings – like today – it takes a lot to drag myself there, but I never regret having gone. I stare at the long vertical crack that's been snaking its way across the ceiling all year. Cracks in the ceiling, like cracks in life, sometimes take a while to appear. I feel like there are cracks creeping open in my body. It's cold. I snuggle up to James for a few more moments of warmth then hurl myself out of bed and close the door on him sleeping deeply behind me. Most mornings go like this. He's nocturnal, stays up late and sleeps well. I fight sleep and lie awake at night and am up early to practise or teach, bumping into things and making a lot of noise as I go. He's either learnt to block out my alarm going off every morning or has become resigned to it. Either way, he never complains.

My body is stiff and my head is already filling up with thoughts. Nothing new there.

I'm tired.
Am I depressed?
My jeans felt tight yesterday
I should call my mum today . . .

I take the train to Charing Cross. Out of the station I turn onto Garrick Street, past the cafes, bookshops and Lamb and Flag pub. I brush away a drunken memory that surfaces from a night there. Smashed pint glass. All of us kicked out. Night out over. I take a sharp left on Rose Street and sprint across Long Acre and into Mercer Street. I've arrived.

The ninety-minute class I go to twice a week is intimate. Most of us recognize one another and, although it hasn't crossed the line into friendship just yet, I like seeing the same faces. The familiarity is an anchor. It reminds me of going to Ashtanga Self-practice spaces where we practise with the same people. We come here for Dharma Yoga, a method developed by Dharma Mittra, a Brazilian. Now in his eighties, Dharma Mittra trained with an Indian guru for a long time before opening the Dharma Yoga Center in New York in 1975. It's a method that focuses deeply on the Eight Limbs, specifically the Yamas and Niyamas. The teacher I practise with talks often about practising compassion and bringing aspects of yoga philosophy into our lives.

I'm drawn to this because I think a lot about modern yoga and how different it is to the practice that emerged in ancient times. When I talk about modern yoga, I mean practices that have emerged since the 1900s. But I also mean yoga and how it relates to our modern lives in the twenty-first century because I'm not against evolution at all. Far from it. We all need a practice that is going to be compatible with the lives we now lead. But I feel the essence of the practice should remain intact.

The old yoga was intended to be about self-discovery and meditation but many of the newer practices we have today don't always appear to adhere to those principles.

I've been to classes where there's so much freestyling in terms of the postures we might do that I've felt disorientated. I prefer order and a sense of formality – without being dogmatic or rigid – for there to be a sense of returning to something on the mat in order to dig deeper. We have to understand the rules even if that means pushing against them and sometimes breaking them to find the path that best suits us. This takes practice, but having a structure is what has paved the way for spiritual work for me and helped take my focus away from the yoga postures themselves when I found myself getting fixated on them. They're fun and make me feel good. They're a comfort too, but they're also meant to be a means to an enlightened future.

It was in this Dharma class, recommended to me by a yoga teacher friend, that I started finding myself again when I first became disillusioned with teaching. Initially I wasn't interested. I didn't much like going to classes where I didn't know the teacher anymore. I avoided yoga fads and didn't want to try anything new. Dharma yoga looked showy from the arm balances that I saw on Instagram and knew I couldn't do, so I was put off. But I lived too far away to travel to my Ashtanga teacher so eventually went along. 'Practise each pose as a prayer' is something my Dharma teacher says regularly.

The first class I went to reduced me to a sweaty dribbling pulp and I couldn't keep up with the pace. There wasn't enough emphasis on synching the breath and the movement (as is the Ashtanga way), which I was confused by because it was so deeply ingrained in the way I practise and teach. Some of the poses made me feel like crying, for at least the first month of going to those classes. I'd arrived with a sore heart after two years of working as a yoga teacher. I felt burnt out, disappointed, angry and bruised. Getting on a yoga mat is the last thing I want to do at times like that. My body almost always feels tight, like it's letting me down. My pelvis is one of the first things to go, hips tight, hamstrings resistant. It feels like everything inside me is bolted together with rusty screws that won't budge. I know my body is saying 'Listen, pay attention!' but I never enjoy facing it when it's doing that. Getting on my mat is usually the only way to make things better.

Back bending is big in this approach to doing yoga postures, and after about ten years of forward folding with Ashtanga, my body wasn't having any of it at first. Our bodies are designed to bend forwards, which is why back bending is so useful but it felt relentless in Dharma. We did very few forward folds and didn't sit down until the end. I was used to Ashtanga, where most of the Primary Series – which is the first sequence – involves forward bends in both standing and seated postures. It's not a perfect sequence, just like no yoga is. One of its flaws is that there is no build-up or preparation before doing wheel pose, which is a back bend that comes towards the end of the Primary Series, but you're only required to do it three times before moving on. So my body hadn't had much experience with moving backwards when I arrived at Dharma yoga.

I've long had an ambivalent relationship with back bends because, although they're hard work, they also have a moreish quality and are quite addictive for me. Once I found a rhythm with them at the Dharma classes I wanted more. I also started learning about the connection between moving in this way and how I was feeling emotionally. My body's willingness to do back bends is often a good sign. It tends to mean I'm feeling emotionally steady and strong or at least am on the mend if I've been dealing with tough emotions. You have to be up for back bending when it involves bursting your heart open like that. This is why I always want to hide away from them when my heart's hurting.

In the Dharma class, turning the spine the other way seemed to creep into almost every posture, as did going upside down with different headstands, handstands, forearm stands. I love inversions but before I arrived at Dharma I could only do headstands comfortably, and so many back bends left me feeling all churned up. I felt like I was uncovering a deep sadness that had been hidden away for a long time, maybe years. This unlocking of buried feelings makes sense because in back bends we're turning our ribcage – the cage of secrets that protects the heart – inside out. Stuck stuff is going to have to come out eventually.

Despite that overwhelming first class, I kept going back. It felt demanding on my body but I craved that. It fed my natural instinct to push myself. I think it's this kind of survivor gene (or stubborn streak) that pulled me through the disordered eating and drinking years. I would have done anything to get rid of food I couldn't contain in my body, as much as I would walk to the furthest off licence that might still be open late at night when I needed a drink. It's that same determination I think that kept bringing me back to yoga when I had given up on it, just to see if it might work again.

Dharma yoga opened my eyes and excited me because we practised postures I'd written off, like the many hand balances. In Ashtanga, traditionally you're not supposed to move further on into the later sequences (there are six in total) until you have mastered the first. Your teacher guides you and lets you know when they think you're ready to add more postures to your repertoire, so I stayed at the same place in the Second Series for a long time. Dharma yoga changed all of that. I started exploring postures from the Second and Third series and over time discovering that some of them were physically within reach. Others required such intense mental stamina to do that I became hooked on that alone because my wayward mind likes nothing more than having something to focus on. It feels like a form of mental training. My teacher pushed me and everyone in the class wherever we might be on our journey. She got me into my first handstand (I still need a wall nearby for reassurance when I do it alone) and helped me into Handstand Scorpion (a crazy balance where you bend your knees and arch your spine in a fascinating way). She cared. I started to feel safe and trust her. That's what I need in a yoga space – to feel safe and seen.

Today I'm sleepy and heavy-limbed, but I'm here, and that's what counts. I'm lying on my stomach when my teacher comes over to help me move deeper into Bow Pose. She inches my right foot closer to my hand as I reach back with every exhale. 'This is impossible,' I tell her, laughing. My neighbours on nearby mats start laughing too. There is joy in this room, in this practice, and this is what keeps me here. About an hour in (several headstands, twists and deep hip openers later) the magic of yoga happens. The discipline present in yoga frequently means being faced with doing something you would rather not. There are poses I'd rather leave out because they're difficult or take too much effort when I'm low on energy. There are others that I do as quickly as I can when the teacher isn't looking because they ask too much and feel wrong (I'm talking about chin stand – urgh). But just as there are no shortcuts in life, there is no way around those poses, only to go through them – in a way that is appropriate for our bodies, of course. I often wonder when I skip things what I might be missing out on. This is how the practice works.

Shortly before the end of class, we lie down and let all effort go. Bodies heavy, sinking into our mats. I imagine gravity pulling my body into the centre of the earth. I sense it dragging all of the physical aches, tightness and emotional heartache away. I feel one of the cracks within me might be willing to let some light in. We all emerge from the practice room, sweat evaporating, muscles fatigued, ponytails unravelled, brains focused. Yoga can be a way toook at oneself. It's also a way for me to distil where I am. It gets my feet back on the ground so that all the thoughts (like wishing I hadn't taken so many wrong turns and wasted years crashing into and burning things in my life) and all the worries about work and money, or getting angry about yoga being too commercial or the usual complaints I have about my own body that preoccupy and drain me – they all lose their power.

In the changing room I take my bag from its locker and resist turning my phone on for as long as possible. Reality can wait a while; I want this balanced feeling to last. I step into the shower feeling achy, sore, alive. The twist in this tale is that my own practice is the only thing that helps me get to know myself, which is how yoga was meant to be. It also helps me step away from the agonizing halo of commercialism that surrounds the yoga industry and helps me see things as they are but not be consumed by them. The questioning, never-ending thinking and analyzing the intricacies of what yoga is or isn't and the constant chatter and misinformation around it are diffused and matter less when I step onto my mat and look within.

I feel calmer.

It's okay.

I love yoga, how could I forget?

CHAPTER 5

Practice is Everything

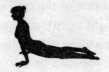

In his book *The Mirror of Yoga*,[13] globally revered Ashtanga teacher Richard Freeman opens with: 'Yoga starts with listening. When we listen, we are giving space to what is.' This sums up what my practice has come to mean to me in recent years. I spent so long feeling disconnected from the practice because of my personal problems that I wasn't capable of listening or digging deeper. I wasn't engaged in a fulfilling practice. I was just getting by. These days yoga for me is all about exploring a relationship – to yourself, to others and how we engage in the world. It's not a religion per se but in many ways it offers hope, direction and a structure that I believe in. I think it's for this reason that yoga complements the lives of many of those who practise a faith.

I've met people who practise yoga and have told me that it helps deepen their relationship with God, which is wonderful, and I can relate. Though I haven't discarded my Muslim roots, I don't follow Islam exclusively. For me, yoga is compatible with Islam, or indeed any faith, and gives me hope that there might be a higher consciousness or something otherworldly out there taking care of the order of things in nature and the cosmos. It took a long time for me to trust this, and yoga makes me keep questioning, but I like having that faith; it feels hopeful. It was the same in ancient times during the Upanishadic and Vedic periods in South Asia. I'll never know for sure what is 'out there' but I feel a greater connection with something outside of myself when I practise and it grips me under the skin. That's enough for me.

Of course, yoga is about so much more than the postures, but I'm a physical person and I need them. I've never been someone who can roll out of bed and sit to meditate. I've tried many times to do that and it doesn't work. I've always been a bad sleeper, which means I often wake up sooner than I would like to, and my head's never empty first thing in the morning. I would much rather roll over and try to get some more sleep but I never can. I've learnt to go with this rather than fight it but instead of leaping out of bed and charging into my day like I used to, I now prefer gazing at the ceiling and letting my body and mind settle into the morning. Then, as thoughtfully as I can, I step into the day.

One of the most important things I've learnt about practice is that it's best approached in a way that's going to ensure that I do it. I'm better suited to moving before sitting in meditation, which is probably why I took to yoga, and specifically Ashtanga yoga, where sitting and then lying down in meditation comes at the end of the sequence. Even on days I don't want to practise – and there are so many of those days – I do it anyway. I might modify what I practice, practise for a shorter time or I may be more distracted but going through the motions is part of my routine. I don't expect miracles or seismic shifts every time I practise, but a form of transformation does usually take place. Sometimes it's subtle and I have to really look for it, which goes back to the idea of listening. Often the impact of my practice can be as simple as carving out some stillness and quiet time before I reach for my phone or open my laptop and let the inevitable noise of the outside world flood in. I've learnt that I'm in with a better chance of having a good day when I take that quiet time every day. As an introvert, I know that I am easily stimulated by conversation, my brain fills with questions and I can't switch off, so I try where I can to take brief moments in the day when I can be quiet – it's as simple as pulling back and not speaking sometimes and can take as little as ten or twenty minutes. Being quiet is like a reset before I plug back in. I don't do it enough because it's so much easier to give it up when I'm busy or having a great time with friends, but I've got better at knowing what my body and mind prefer.

This hasn't always been the case. I was an all-or-nothing person with practice for a long time because I was an all-or-nothing person with everything else I did for most of my life. It didn't help that I had chosen to follow Ashtanga, which is traditionally meant to be a six-day-a-week practice (apart from new and full moon days, when you get a rest). I followed the rules for many years, then slipped and felt I was failing when I didn't manage it. This was a heavy burden for a long time, but it also fed my need to burn off some of the damage of binging during the bulimia years. I was being sick every day and didn't like exercise classes, so yoga was a way to keep me moving and allow me to purge in another way. It wasn't until I stopped drinking and when I got bored of the hot yoga that got me through the early days of sobriety that I felt able to give myself permission to return to Ashtanga and practise how it might best suit me. This means I don't stick to the traditional rules anymore and most importantly I'm not riddled with guilt.

The way I teach Ashtanga too is informed by my practice. I follow 'the rules' and teach according to the traditional sequence but the people who come to my classes arrive in different bodies and in various emotional states. I see who is in front of me and I adapt accordingly. According to Ashtanga tradition, you're not supposed to move to the next posture until you've mastered the one before it and your teacher tells you when you're ready. This makes sense to a degree because the sequence is designed in an order that prepares the body for the next posture as you go along. But it also takes away the autonomy of yoga being your own practice. There are some poses I know I might never be able to do because my skeleton isn't made for it (foot behind the head, for example). There are other postures that come later that my body likes (the complicated headstands and arm balances) and my mind craves the concentration required to do them. The same will go for students in my classes. I watch them move, I assess the data and we go from there. It also means we have fun. It's important that we're doing a strong practice in my classes and staying focused (distraction is a big symptom of modern life), but I want people to enjoy the practice too and look forward to coming, which is probably me projecting my own stuff in response to the days I hated going to classes.

In many ways I don't mind if I'm not the most dedicated with yoga postural practice itself all the time. I try to be because I get so much out of it but, after all those years of what felt like a competition with myself to push and pull my body into complicated poses and beating myself up when I didn't make it, I've made my peace with it now. The practice was a reflection of how I approached everything else in my life: impulsively, impatiently and without compassion. I was taking everything too seriously and the pressure was too much.

I don't want practice to be a chore anymore, I want to love it, so I had to find a way to make that possible. The truth is that I don't feel that pressure now and I truly believe that some days sitting and staring out of the window, moving through a short sequence of postures and then sitting to meditate is better for me than pushing myself, which I can easily default to if I don't keep an eye on myself. Our bodies are wise (wiser than our minds, I'd say) and they don't lie. It took me a long time to understand that. My head loves practising complicated twisty, bendy, binding and folding postures but I'm learning to listen (which is a slow process, in my experience) when the body is saying no.

Freeman's idea of listening involves paying attention as much as possible. A way I find helpful to do this is to ask myself *what is my body telling me?* as I move through a series of postures on my mat. Doing this keeps me from trying to fall into the old pattern of forcing my body into shapes it might not want to do. I extend this approach in the way I teach too, reminding students that we're all doing a version of the posture. I'm there to guide and lead the way as the teacher but it's the students' job to work out what's most appropriate for them.

Another reason my relationship with yoga has been changing is because, although the practice has been the thing that has sustained me most of my life, I have also learnt so many lessons in life in other places, like the recovery fellowships, through many Buddhist practices and in therapy. All these paths complement each other. Also, somewhere along the line I've developed a relationship with what I call my Acceptance Muscle. It's a metaphor I use for trying to strengthen an important aspect of life that I've struggled with for so many years. I still don't always find accepting what life throws at me simple, but practising acceptance of where

I am on my mat has helped me cultivate an ability to apply it to other areas of my life. It's all too easy for me to look back on my life and lament and feel sorrow for the years of pain I felt. Sometimes they feel like years wasted when I could have been happier. Thinking that way makes me blame myself for missing out on the normative life benchmarks: buying a home, getting married, having children. While I still don't know if I wanted all of these things, I can end up thinking I've messed things up and am left feeling sad. The only way out of this thought process is to tell myself that none of what has happened matters. Where I am now does, and I have to learn to accept that and try not to judge it in order to find peace.

I spent so long thinking something was wrong with me, searching for labels, a diagnosis, anything to explain why I hurt myself so much with drinking and food and destructive relationships, but I've let that go now. I talk to a great therapist and none of our work is about pathologizing me, but simply talking, analyzing, piecing together, finding words for feelings. I think of the therapeutic process like Kintsugi, which is the Japanese art of putting broken pottery pieces back together with gold. The philosophy behind the practice is that through embracing flaws and imperfections, you can create an even stronger, more beautiful piece of art. We're all miracles and artworks in our own ways. We're all made differently, whether we're able-bodied, disabled, emotionally stable or mentally ill. That's where the practice comes in – to help us find a way that works for us and to use it to understand who we are behind the different versions of ourselves and the roles and responsi-bilities we have in our lives.

For someone like me with obsessive tendencies, practising acceptance has felt like a healthier approach. I think it makes me better at teaching yoga too. I wish I had got to that earlier. It's so easy for me to get wrapped up in self-absorption but when I step onto my mat it becomes a place for showing up and a place to discover. It's an opportunity to remind myself that I probably spend a lot of time telling myself stories about how my life's going. How I should do better and work harder, wondering what's wrong with me that led to so many of my relationships ending. I know I've lost perspective, and regurgitating ideas like that until my head is filled with them isn't going to do much good.

I know that the practice helps and I'm better off with it, but I don't think doing more hours of it through gritted teeth makes for a better experience. It's important for there to be joy in it, and listening to my body and responding as I move through the practice on my mat allows me to take what I discover into the rest of my day. It helps me remember to take deeper breaths when I'm anxious in a crowded place and to remember to be as compassionate as I can with someone who might have pissed me off. This gets easier when I'm practising how to do it with myself.

At the same time, I know that I need to be physical or my mood will start to drop. I know that I'll become anxious and not know why, which risks other things going wrong. Food might start becoming hard to navigate, my desire to see people usually starts to fall away, until slowly there's nothing left but me and a load of misery. Three days away from practice is the limit for me. I know I've got to turn things around pretty fast if I let it get that far. Sometimes I'll let things wane and if it gets to two weeks, I'm in a danger zone because I know it'll take a lot to get me back. But once I stop lecturing myself for letting this happen, all that's left is to get over myself and face the mat.

For me practice is now about doing something regularly and going deeper over time. As with any habit, we get better and stronger at what we do more of. But practice is not something I've been naturally good at most of my life. As a child I hated practising the piano, and my teacher would despair each week when it was obvious I hadn't done my homework. During the drinking years and when I was stuck in binge–purge cycles every day, the constant attack on my body meant I wasn't progressing or getting stronger physically or spiritually. I didn't have a solid practice because in a sense I was fighting it with my other behaviours even if I felt I had no choice. I think practice only really works if you want to do it and if you're consistent and make it a priority, which I was only able to learn when I wasn't drinking or making myself sick every day.

When I started teaching yoga, I spent a long while finding my feet, teaching how I thought I was supposed to and feeling all the pressures and pains of having to come up with elaborate choreography, devise enigmatic playlists and dressing in a certain way. As I gained more experience, my confidence grew and once again my own practice showed me the way. I remember meditating in a headstand at the end of practice one day and I started thinking. I realized that none of the stuff I had got caught up in mattered. The bigger question should be: how could I share the spirit of the practice as I experienced it in my teaching and let students discover things their own way? It changed the entire course of my teaching from then on, and I was happier because I was teaching what I practised, which feels like the right place to be teaching from.

Whatever your practice might be, I think it only works when you start to make it your own. To me, sharing the spirit of the practice means explaining that idea of observation, of presence; sometimes it's having a chat after class with someone and showing them how they might arrange their bodies to sit tall for meditation. It's sharing things I do in public places when I'm anxious on public transport in case that might help. It's also doing my best to lead by example and for me that means revealing my flaws, talking about aspects of yoga I find hard, and where I've come from and the fact that I'm not getting it right all the time. One of the biggest misconceptions I came across through working in yoga was that some people seemed to think I knew everything there is to know about yoga. But of course I don't, I'm still working everything out like we all are. That's why I love the practice; it keeps me learning.

One of the big things yoga has taught me in the twenty-five or so years since I first stepped on (and off and on) a mat is that happiness/wellness/contentment doesn't lie in a more flexible body (even though it feels pretty good when that starts to happen). It's actually to be found in discipline and doing something with dedication and consistency to gain a profound understanding of ourselves. This work takes time – years or a lifetime. It can be painful, and sometimes presents us with ugly or harsh realities. But this is also what I think living a truthful life entails. I think the same applies whatever your practice or faith might be if yoga isn't your way.

Another thing that unexpectedly taught me something about yoga was running. I discovered running by accident two weeks before my fortieth birthday. I was feeling flat and, to change things up, I did something I've only done a handful of times: I went for a jog. In the dark – so no one would see me. I've never liked running. I found its repetitiveness boring, and the intense cardio made me anxious. But I put on some drum'n'bass in my headphones to distract me and help pretend it wasn't happening and off I went. I ran and walked to a nearby common. One foot in front of the other, gathering momentum. Slowly I started getting a feeling of purpose.

So I did it again. The more I did, the quieter the music got. It was hard work for a long time before I saw any progress. Then one day I noticed that I had run for the length of the fifteen-minute track that I was listening to and that's when it hit me for the first time. For so many years, practice had been about pushing myself. Hurling myself out of bed at 5 a.m. to get to a studio before going to work, traipsing around London, pounding Sun Salutations on mats around the city searching for ninety minutes of peace. That day on my run I realized that I wanted my practice to be less about chasing and more about building something. I had been here before. Just stay sober for the day, fellow recoverists would tell me when I said I couldn't do it. One day at a time adds up. It's the same with practice. Building not chasing had to be the way forward. Running taught me one of the best lessons I've learnt about what yoga now means to me.

Listening to the Body

We're all going to have different relationships with our bodies, and I sometimes still struggle with mine. Although yoga means so much more to me than the postures alone, I couldn't do without them. Before yoga, I had tried so hard to get into exercise, but my motive wasn't about feeling good back then; it was a form of punishment on my body. Yoga offered something different. That early discovery I made at those YMCA classes as a teenager showed me that exploring my body in a new way worked for me. I fell in love with those strange shapes that had felt awkward at first and sometimes made me laugh. I started to enjoy moving in an unfamiliar way and finding out what was going on in my body. Not a lot has changed decades later. I still love twists, the initial impossibility of hand balances, back bends and binds, where you wrap an arm around a calf or thigh to grab the other wrist from behind. Making these shapes, focusing on alignment and form, helps focus my mind. I see that intense focus in others when I practise in a room with them. Practising in a group is a beautiful and precious thing. When we come together in a room, breathing and moving together, synching and falling out of synch with our separate breaths, there's a tangible power that you can't recreate alone. Like electricity, there's a spark, a life force that connects you all, and that collective energy – a power greater than ourselves – is what moves us and holds us together. You can't capture that in a photograph. No picture ever reflects what's truly going on.

We all carry stories in our bodies, of the good and bad things that have happened to us. I'm fascinated by how much pain we can cart through life for years without paying attention. The postures have helped me learn more about what my body is holding onto in a way that nothing else has. My body wasn't made for yoga poses. I'm not naturally flexible so my body is like an elastic band. Sometimes it is stretchy and willing – those are the days I enjoy the most – but at other times all my muscles feel taut, warning me I might snap something if I argue with them too much. Days like this are disappointing but also a big lesson in patience. There are aches and pains that I have only started paying attention to in recent years. My right shoulder is especially tight, as are my hips. It's only since I introduced the idea of listening into my practice that I started watching what was going on in my body rather than trying to force it to do something it might never want to.

The postures also show me how to teach. To be compassionate with the bodies of people who come to my classes, I know I have to do it with myself first. I remember someone coming to speak to me at a class I taught for staff at a charity. She told me that the words I used during the group's resting time at the end of their practice resonated, which was lovely to hear. I had talked about 'feeling the earth has got your back, trusting it will hold you'. I told the student that the words that came out when I was teaching were never planned and always came from my own struggles. I remember feeling weary when I taught that class. I was going through a period of heartbreak at the time and noticed I was talking about the heart a lot in my classes. At some point I'd usually ask everyone to see if they could allow their hearts to rest, hearts that have seen it all, been through so much. I realized through teaching that I was becoming more of a heart person than a thinky head person. It felt like a good way to go.

I'm not sure how but there's an uncanny way this practice helps me find and hold onto faith when I've lost it. That said, I know it's not for everyone. Yoga is one way for spiritual growth but it's not the only way. I have tried many other approaches at times when yoga didn't feel like it was enough. If I had found another path that worked better, I might have replaced yoga with something else entirely.

In the early noughties I found myself looking longingly at congregations outside churches from the top deck of buses. I'd watch huge groups of devotees chatting outside mosques and I'd want what they had: belonging, shared belief and complete trust in the method. So when a friend who attended a monthly chanting group hosted by Hare Krishnas in Covent Garden invited me along, I went. Everyone was lovely, the food was tasty, and I had a good time. But it wasn't hitting the spot I was looking for.

Some time after that, in 2010, a friend and I went to a summer festival. It was an alcohol- and drug-free event inspired by Western Buddhist principles. I had wanted to go because I thought that living among fields in the sunshine without any alcohol for a few days would kickstart me towards sobriety. We Londoners, who had never had the money to go to a festival before, turned up ill-equipped wearing Converse trainers and leather jackets. It rained for all five days we were there, so I was perpetually cold and there was definitely mud in my knickers. I still loved it. My inner hippie was emancipated as I danced barefoot on grass in 5Rhythms workshops, cried in Shamanic drumming circles and stood naked under the stars in an outdoor shower cubicle. I felt a rebirthing was taking place. But it wasn't meant to be because I went home and started drinking again. I loved that place though and returned for many years without fail. And then I stopped. I don't know if the festival got worse or I got better but that last year, walking around as a volunteer steward, I saw with fresh eyes some things I had noticed previously but had been too wrapped up in myself to question. I saw all the usual festival fare: white women wearing sari tops and bindis, and stalls selling clothes and homewares from Nepal and Tibet. That hadn't been enough to bother me before. What did stick out this time was that there seemed to be more public displays of nakedness. On one hand I thought I should live and let live, but on the other it seemed to give a sexualized 'free love' vibe to the festival, which might have been why a bloke I'd met in a coffee queue the previous day danced over to me in a 5Rhythms workshop and told me to take my dress off. That hadn't happened before. I frowned at him and danced away, leaving him with a bemused look on his face as though what he'd demanded was a reasonable thing to have done.

My steward partner and I saw a sign outside a tent for a tribal markings workshop on one of our walkarounds. I stuck my head around the tent door and saw dancing bodies covered in paint. Something didn't feel right about that. There was also a Native American Sweat Lodge at the festival. I've no idea if it was run by a Native American – it may well have been. But I felt uncomfortable thinking that it quite possibly wasn't. Questions about cultural appropriation and appreciation started firing off in my mind. Which was it that was going on here? I also saw people passing a secret bottle of wine around as we sat by a fire late one evening. There were rules about drinking to make the festival inclusive, and as a person attempting recovery that made me angry.

Maybe I was wrong to feel weird. But everything I was seeing this time, coupled with the fact that there were very few people of colour every year, was starting to feel odd. It wasn't just me who was in two minds about the nudity I was seeing either. A sex addict who I met in the recovery meeting tent told me he had attended to feel safe but he was now relapsing as a result of seeing so many bare breasts. I wasn't into seeing the occasional man walking around with his genitals out either. I asked my friend who had gone to the festival with me the very first time what she thought: 'It's an issue of consent. I wasn't expecting everyone to be naked in the sauna. It was the first time I've sat next to a strange man with his penis out. And it's not consensual when I see them naked in fields either. That wouldn't be allowed at any other festival so why there?'

I saw her point. Most people looked like they were having a great time, as I had done many times myself, but it all suddenly felt more oppressive than about freedom. I've never been back.

But I've never stopped searching for spirituality in my life, and discovering yoga has never stopped me seeking solace in other places. Perhaps it's been out of a fear of committing to a single process and doing things wrong. If I dabbled and didn't claim I was a devout follower of anyone's method, I could cop out when I wanted to. Or maybe – and I think this is most likely – I'm just not made for one single practice. I've dabbled with so many different routes to find peace that I've ended up with a hybrid approach to life. There are traces of Islam in my belief system hanging around from where everything started for me at home as a child. It's why I can't stop myself saying *Inshallah* (God willing) and *Mashallah* (what God has willed) because it's part of the fabric of who I have been for so long. It's why I'm still moved by the call to prayer when I'm in Muslim countries. It's also why I draw from the many wisdoms I learnt in the recovery fellowships and from yoga philosophy, Western philosophies and Zen Buddhism as well as people I've met and spent time with. So I wonder whether the method for practice matters at all so long as it's personal, has meaning and works for you. Surely that's the most important thing? This is why I believe there's no one right way to practise yoga. I've practised for long enough to know this to be true, and my way of yoga has changed so much during that time. It feels important to be flexible and compassionate with ourselves in our approach and I think all of that starts with listening. Above all, the most important thing is to find a way to practise that works and (although I know I wasn't very good at this for a long time) to keep doing it.

Alienated Awareness
and Dropping the Bass with the Zen

I must have had hundreds of conversations over the years with one of my closest friends, Stuart, about what practice means to him. We met twelve years ago at the alcohol-free festival the first summer I went. A practising Buddhist in the Zen tradition, Stuart isn't an official teacher, which he's always keen to remind me of whenever I go to him filled with questions. He's always keen to make clear that he's talking to me about his own practice and that I shouldn't treat him as an authority. But I've learnt so much from Stuart that this book wouldn't be complete without his frank and honest words in it.

Stuart has been practising Zen through the teachings of Thích Nhất Hạnh (known as Thay) for more than twenty years. Thay – whose teachings have had a profound impact on my life, too – passed away at midnight on 22nd January 2022. He was aged 95 and in Vietnam where he began practising as a monk. Stuart found Zen when he was newly in recovery from drug addiction so he knows a thing or two about what turning your life around involves. His unflinching approach to practice inspires me because he lives it, dedicating himself to and embodying the practice in a way that I can only hope for myself one day. He's not perfect by any means. Far from it. I know his flaws and we argue and disagree on many things, but he has also taken care of me when I've needed it. And he knows how to use a swear word, which makes me feel at home.

Stuart has a way of turning up when I need him. When I'm depressed, I prefer to hide away. At those times he'll nudge me out for a walk or take me for a ride on his motorbike. It always helps. Sometimes the only way to get the heart and mind to shift is to take the body itself on a journey to a different place. One weekend we rode to Greenwich Park and as we climbed the hill to take in the view across the city, I was blathering on about the disillusioning things that led to me writing this book. Stuart seemed to be having his own crisis about the state of Buddhism in the West.

Mindfulness has become an industry that has nothing to do with Buddhism. What we're talking about with this practice is eternity and everything. This practice is about fundamentally changing your whole way of being and experiencing the world. It's not an add-on to make life a bit better around the edges.

'You're saying that mindfulness isn't something to cram into your lunch break?' I asked him.

'Exactly, because this practice is so radical, it can't fit into that frame at all. It just won't work as it's meant to.'

Though I've read many of Thích Nhất Hạnh's books and attended a Zen group at certain points in my life, most of what I've learnt about Zen is through talking and practising with Stuart himself. I'm not an expert on Zen matters, nor a Buddhist, but I draw inspiration and practice from this tradition because the Five Mindfulness Trainings (guidance for living life, similar to the Eight Limbs) are so practical and easy to follow. I learnt from Stuart that the Buddha lived around 500 BCE. As far as we know the Buddha suffered a great deal and much of what he did was a rejection of modern life. His motivation to practise was seeking an answer to one of life's big questions: *in a world full of inevitable sadness, how do we find peace?* I asked Stuart what his own practice had taught him about that. He explained:

The Buddha thought modern life was empty, we're all going to die so we should consider what is of value in life. He pushed his experience right to the end. And in a modern context, if someone in his condition turned up and said, 'I want to do mindfulness,' he'd probably say, 'You need to go and do a therapeutic process first because you're too far out there, and it might be dangerous.' Because what we're actually looking for in this practice is an escape from normal life. It's not a soft thing to help you fit in with modern life and put up with it. It's about finding solutions to that.

We generate sad thoughts and a sense of self which is going to die. We worry about what's going to happen in the future. This is an imaginary world we create in our heads. We have an opinion on the government, we worry about our health or what kind of wallpaper we want. All these things are imagined but we treat them as if they were real. And the practice is about immersing ourselves in the miracle of the moment.

It sounded to me as though Stuart was talking about mindfulness as being a form of mental training, a commitment and discipline, much like yoga. I've met many people with austere practices and dogmatic teachers on my own yoga journey, and often it seems to be missing the point to think of any practice as a gruelling process with the idea that if you work hard one day, you'll be happy one day. I asked Stuart what he thought.

We should ask ourselves what we mean by happiness, because we confuse happiness and peace of mind with pleasure, and it's not. There's something deeper than that, which is actually a peace really. You can be doing a yoga class, and doing some-

thing very difficult and demanding and right on that edge, but if you're totally in it, that's joy. We have quite a harsh idea of discipline. In the gym, some people might be working out to the point that they're going to throw up. If you're disturbed in your mind and you're pushing through, I'd say that's the wrong kind of discipline. But with yoga you can really be going for it, but you're conscious and your mind is calm and you're staying with it. So having self-discipline isn't really it. I think you need a certain peace within it. I'd say you'd be happier doing that than sitting at home with a beer and watching Netflix. Yoga is about learning to be with discomfort and being at peace with it, which is much the same in Zen.

Stuart knows a thing or two about discipline. He came to Zen in his late thirties when his life was falling apart. Trying to escape a strict Protestant upbringing had resulted in him taking drugs from the age of fifteen, living in squats and a life of misery ensued. He was attracted to the warrior ethos of the Samurai – twelfth-century military officers from early-modern Japan – and was drawn to the hope that Zen offered. He says:

I came to Zen when I was in ruins. Finding Zen was about finding meaning and connection with other people. But it is also a form of training. If you apply it, you'll achieve peace and a better perspective within a few months, and be better able to deal with your life. But to go deeper, it takes years. It took me years because I was a thug really. I had spent all of my life around hard men and it takes practice to find the softness.

My experience is that men like to be hard. And in a way, it's easy because you cut off your emotions and you don't care about anything. You end up having a thick skin and you're willing to fight with people. If you take someone like

Thích Nhất Hạnh and what he lived through in the Vietnam
War: he never gave in to hatred, and he was still at peace.
He saw his friends die and he didn't take sides in that war.
A lot of Vietnamese hated Americans. He didn't.

'How has Thay done it?' I asked.

He applied the practice from an early age. He said, 'The
temptation to give in to hatred may be there and the easiest
thing would be to pick up a gun and shoot these people but
we can't do that.' He meant that it's not negotiable in our
tradition, because there's always a better way. However much
harder it is to let go of the hate, you do it for a better world
and for your own peace. For me that was just: wow, bang!
Because being a junkie and with all that misery and hatred
that I'd grown up with, it was just a normal thing that people
did. And then you meet him, and you hear his life story, and
you think, 'Oh, there's hope.' He embodies the Buddha. It
was like dropping the bass with the Zen and my life was
never the same again.

As Stuart and I stood at the viewing point at the top of the
hill, I remembered something he had mentioned before about
how the practice can go wrong. He described it as 'alienated
awareness'. I asked him to explain that more fully.

It's a thing where your practice can be very cold, so you'll be
deeply present, but there's no heart in it. So if you've got a
very serious strict meditation practice, you might be able to
focus your mind and you can be present in the moment, but
you haven't cultivated any joy. We meditate with our bodies,
not with our minds. Some people find it difficult to meditate

*because they haven't experienced their bodies. So yoga or
martial arts or sports really adds to a person's ability to meditate. But if all you've ever done is a sedentary job, and you've
never done much exercise, there's no real way in.*

'So what's the best way to practise?' I asked him.

*In traditional Zen, practice isn't regarded as an intellectual
process. It's a physiological observation. If you sit still, relaxed
and upright and you put your attention on something – you'll
stop thinking. It's as simple as that. So the breath's a good
thing for your attention. Sometimes I like listening to rain
outside; or it could be a pain in your toe. It can be anything
to immerse yourself in so that you're not ruminating.*

Given both of our troubled pasts and my strong belief in the
power of psychotherapy, I wondered what Stuart thought about
that. Surely there had to be a place where practice ended and
therapy began. Or perhaps they were linked, which I feel to
be the case for me.

*Yes and no. Someone who's deeply traumatized or ill will
probably need to go through a therapeutic process. But my
own experience of Western therapy is that it isn't always
successful on its own. It has a place, but there's a Buddhist
approach to this too that is equally valuable, which is about
just being with someone and listening. There's quite a significant overlap in what effective therapy is and what effective
practice is and how you are with people. I don't see that
they're entirely separate. These are universal skills that we
can learn in terms of how to be present with someone, listen
with care, not judge and be open.*

I stared at the skyline and we stood together identifying London landmarks: Canary Wharf, St Paul's Cathedral, the London Eye and the Shard. I tried to be present, in that moment, observing the architecture, aware of being with my friend, listening to the chatter around us, but without giving it lots of meaning. It wasn't easy to do.

'Do you ever get fed up with the practice?' I asked Stuart, thinking about my own walk-outs on yoga.

I have done. I've had little frustrations like, 'why do we do this?' or, 'I don't like that chant,' or, 'the way we do certain things is a waste of time.' But increasingly, I don't think about those things. It's about having confidence in the broader process as a whole and realizing there will always be little niggling things, but actually knowing that this works. Realizing that there's a deeper truth, which is beyond this particular practice, which is in many religions and spiritual traditions or approaches to life, and just believing in that.

'What does practice mean to you?' I asked Stuart.

It means I want to feel at peace, and I want to live my days with joy and ease. There are various factors of enlightenment. There's diligence, mindfulness, paying attention to your experience, there's concentration and letting go. There's the eight-fold path, and the four noble truths. If your life has those things, well, that's what a Buddha or enlightened person is. But also, those are the things to do, the things to cultivate, that will make your life worthwhile.

That felt so profound because Stuart came to the practice when life wasn't worth living.

I think for a lot of people, their lives aren't really worth living. If our lives are filled with misery, as mine was, there's no point being alive, but we have choices. We're born into this universe, where every moment is an absolute miracle beyond our comprehension. It sounds wacky, but if we stop and look around, it's mind-blowing. There are no limits to the practice. One of the monks said the other day that even if you're in a hospital dying you still have the basis of being happy because you're alive.

'Even if you might die?' I asked.

'Even if you're dying,' Stuart said. 'Sounds harsh, but people die peacefully in the worst of conditions. Because if they live that way, they can die that way.'

Hearing Stuart say this made such sense. It blew my mind, to tell the truth. The idea that living a peaceful life could mean dying a peaceful death. What more could any of us want? It sounded like the most powerful incentive I had ever heard to stay close to my practice above everything else and to continue Thay's practice and legacy. For what it can offer me personally, but also in terms of how I interact with and impact the world.

I hoped and trusted in my heart that Thay had died a peaceful death. But it felt like a huge loss for the world. I was sad he was gone. 'It does feel like a certain loneliness now,' Stuart said. 'There's only one thing he would have wanted and that's for us to live each day being the very best human we can. As he always tried to do.'

Where Hope Comes From

It comes from having something to believe in. If you believe in it, it exists. It's believing when there's nothing there. No proof, just blind faith. It's realizing that you're not falling apart even when it feels like you are. It's remembering that you've lived through enough to know that, as the poet Rilke wrote, 'no feeling is final' and therefore all emotions – however despairing – will pass.

Hope is living with ambivalence but deciding that it's time to move forward. Toward somewhere, anywhere. It's looking at trees and finally noticing the beauty in living things that was always there. You couldn't see it for a while because the baggage of pain you've been carrying had become too heavy. But it's time to put those bags down. They don't belong to you anymore. So what can you do?

Look ahead.

Look up.

Hope is staring at the sky and seeing again that there's a force out there bigger than you. It's believing that you will turn a corner – it's just a question of when. Even if you wish that corner was here right now, in this moment – it's trusting that it will come soon.

It's doing whatever it takes and that might mean trying a lot of different things until you find the one that fits. Hope is a choice. It's rolling out your yoga mat if only to step on it to remind yourself that practice is always there. It's going through the motions of a few postures or sitting to gaze out of the window. It's dancing around the room to music that gives you energy. It's walking, with purpose, on busy, noisy streets late at night because that might be what you need.

It's running when you've never been a runner and don't know if you can. But you put on your headphones and pull on your trainers. You walk, run, walk, run. One foot in front of the other slow, fast, faster. You're running just to remind yourself that you have a heart that can beat fast.

Tugging at your sleeves because it's a January night in London and your fingers hurt from the cold. It starts raining, your face is hard from the icy air, you keep going. Snot starts dribbling towards your upper lip. You wipe it away but there's more, dribbling down your mouth. You leave it there and keep running. You turn at the top of the hill, smashing the glistening pavement with each strike, foot to concrete.

Yes legs, yes head, yes heart; keep going.

The music changes: 'Says' by Nils Frahm too loud in your ears, and you know this piece of music so well. It's coming up to 7.03 minutes when the track changes, at that bit that always possesses you, those familiar chords that will forever clutch your heart. A wave of fresh strength floods your body: legs pounding, buckling, feet clambering forwards. You might trip and fall; it doesn't matter.

Because now it feels like you'll never stop running. You run urgently, like the wind because you are the wind. You have become the rain. That bigger-than-you thing in the sky, among the trees, it's back inside you too now and you're running wildly like an animal that has been caged for too long. You feel like you could run for ever or until there's no run left, because that's what you're doing right now.

Your throbbing heart feels like it will burst out of your chest, taking with it the entire gamut of everything that's piled up inside you. Every scrap of disappointment, those years of unanswered pain gushing out, like a dam has broken and joy, euphoria, hope is filling its place. You know this moment won't last but you can't feel broken anymore because you're not. You are here. And you'll remember this next time you have to scrape yourself off the floor again.

Your face is wet with rain, and snot and tears. There's no stopping now. The hope is in your legs, it's in your flesh, heart, bones. It's in your short fast breath. The music stops. You stand still, solid as a mountain under the thick black sky, panting.

This is hope. It's all you've ever needed. Who knows if it'll stick around, but it's down to you to keep looking for it. That's the job. And you've found another place to look next time you lose it again.

CHAPTER 6

The Problem with Gurus

There is a saying that a teacher arrives when the student is ready. I've been lucky to have crossed paths with some great teachers on my yoga journey. Some of them I met and practised with so briefly that they will never know the impact they had. Others, like Gingi, taught me how to teach long before I underwent any formal yoga teacher training. When I turned up at his studio in a drunken haze in 2008, I saw him as a beacon of hope and a reason to climb out of the gutter I felt stuck in. He represented someone who might restore me to sanity. I didn't know it at the time, but he must have sensed what was up with me because he was quick to take himself off that pedestal. He had a gifted way of cultivating intimacy with each of his students but maintaining enough distance. This approach has worked for me too.

When it came to my own teaching, I was so insecure initially that there wasn't any space for inflating my ego. When I eventually came to enjoy teaching, I saw it as an extension of my own relationship with yoga. I think staying close to your own practice as a teacher is important because I've seen too many yoga teachers, spiritual leaders and so-called healers fall from grace after being caught exploiting their positions of power and behaving badly. The power dynamic of leading a group seems to go to their heads, so I wouldn't put your yoga teacher on a pedestal – it never ends well. The best ones, and by that I mean those who have clear boundaries about what's appropriate in their relationship with you, wouldn't want you to anyway. Sadly, this kind of professionalism doesn't always play itself out in the yoga world.

So what makes a great yoga teacher? There's a big danger of turning yoga teachers into celebrities. I think this is a risk because some of them will believe the hype. It also seems at odds with the ethics of yoga itself. These days, greatness is too often bestowed upon teachers who have huge social media followings, those whose bodies can bend into complicated yoga postures and others who are known for inventive sequencing and funky playlists. But in my view, the best teachers tend to be the quieter ones – simply decent, also-flawed human beings. These are the ones I relate to and it's how I tried to be myself when I started teaching. Sadly, the shouty majority who constantly post pictures of themselves doing inaccessible postures most of us can only dream of achieving have come to define the contemporary image of yoga. I'm not suggesting that looking up to any of these influencer yoga types who inspire you is a bad thing, but I think it's good to keep a level head where we can. This is critical when it comes to teachers we meet in real life where it's important not to give all our power away.

Why do some of us put so much faith in gurus? Why have I? For me it fed a desire for reassurance that I was on the right path at times when I didn't trust myself. It's as if I had an unconscious need for a parental figure to offer love and safety on my yoga path, when in fact I should have been learning how to parent and trust myself. I've put too much faith in yoga teachers and healers at difficult points in my life and sadly I wasn't treated with respect. It's in situations like this, when gurus abuse their power, that everyone's in trouble. This is important to talk about because huge scandals of sexual abuse have emerged in the yoga world in recent years.

I can tell my own share of horror stories when it comes to being touched without consent. By men I don't know on nights out, on public transport and that time a coked-up stranger slipped his hand between my legs while I was reaching for a glass from a top shelf at a house party in Brighton. If you're a woman reading this, the chances are you have your own stories of uninvited touch too. This is the insidious patri-archy at work – where men believe it is their right to touch a woman's body without her permission. It happens. I live for a day that it doesn't. Meantime, it's not something you expect to be going on inside yoga spaces.

Some Bad Gurus I've Encountered

The Shaman

For my thirtieth birthday I treated myself to a Shamanic healing session with a man a friend recommended. I had hoped it might be life-changing and quash my desire to drink alcohol, which had started to become a big problem a few years earlier. It was a deeply powerful experience, but also a blur so I don't remember much more than shaking and crying uncontrollably – A LOT. After two hours of that I was physically drained. My muscles ached as if I had done a full-body work-out. I took a bus home, ate a bowl of takeaway ramen and went to bed without drinking. It didn't last and I was back on the bottle the following day.

The Shaman recommended we stay in touch as that was an important part of the after-care he offered. He checked in with me often and slowly I started opening up about my life. I told him that I felt disoriented and emotionally jumbled up several weeks after the session, which he said was part of the process. I suggested it might have something to do with the fact that I couldn't stop drinking red wine. He then told me that drinking red wine, which had a 'high vibration', was my way of trying to connect with my own psychic energy. But I didn't care about being psychic, I just wanted to stop drinking. I was disappointed that his Shamanism hadn't worked. One evening during a phone call where he was teaching me a breathing technique to access the psychic part of me that might cure me, he offered to come over to practise together in person. I was an idiot with no boundaries and let him. Everything was going well until he told me my sexual energy was blocked. He suggested I sit on his lap to open it up and I thought *Woahhhhh, it's time to stop.* It took me a long time to work out what had happened there. Had I let it get that far? Was it my fault? Of course it wasn't. When you ask someone for help, that's not how things should go. I never heard from him again.

The Indian Warrior
The worst experience I had with a guru was in India three years after I met the Shaman. I had ended up in Kerala after being persuaded to go by a yoga teacher I didn't know very well who was running a teacher training course there. I was in bad physical and emotional shape and still drinking at the time but had high hopes. In India I would learn discipline, develop a solid practice and return home renewed. I had a lot of faith in the power of what can happen in India. I'm not the only one. It's a country that gets romanticized all the time.

Yoga teachers love telling us they're travelling to India when what they really mean is that they are going to a resort in Goa. It's a wonderful tourist hotspot and every time I've been to India I go there for a rest because, although India has captivated my heart for many years, it's a vast country that can also be exhausting mainly due to sexual harassment. I have had my boobs groped on the sleeper train from Goa to Bombay and in the streets of Delhi. There was that time a hostel worker grabbed my jet-lagged friend's arm and tried to kiss her while the rest of us were napping. As the only Hindi speaker in the group (I speak Urdu but it sounds similar), I ran down to reception livid and shouting while the workforce made up entirely of men laughed at us.

When I went to undertake the teacher training in Kerala, I was about to embark on something that ended in a disaster. Amanda, a Californian I met out there who became my roommate, was the best part of that trip. I wouldn't have survived it without her. There were five of us on the course and it started going wrong very quickly. The teacher who had invited me had a meltdown and left so the resort owner, who I'll call B, took over. B, who looked like a mythological Indian warrior with his billowing trousers and thick curly ponytail, took a shine to Amanda and was dismissive of me. I couldn't work out why. I studied and practised hard, hoping he would change his mind about me. He did, but not in a way I was expecting.

As part of our training, we were each given a *Panchakarma* treatment, which in Sanskrit means 'five actions'. These are a series of Ayurvedic massages designed to purify the body. Ayurveda is an ancient system of natural medicine, which I've long found fascinating even if I don't always follow the lifestyle guidance it offers. I felt awkward about being massaged by B because something just didn't feel right about him, but

I was vulnerable and in need of major spiritual cleaning, so I stuck it out. Things eventually went wayward when B said my sexual energy was blocked during a treatment. *Here we go again*, I thought. *Another spiritual guru telling me I'm sexually messed up. This seems to be turning into a pattern in my life.* He said a vaginal enema would be my only cure. *Hang on, what?!* 'Who would administer such a procedure?' I asked, lying naked and glistening in various oils beneath a thin sheet. It would be him, he said. Naturally, I refused, and things went from weird to worse.

One evening, our group took a post-dinner promenade in a nearby tea plantation where B told me that he was in love with me and had fantasized about sleeping with me. I was shocked and asked him to stop saying these uncomfortable things, but it seemed that the more I resisted his sexual advances the bolder he became. I wanted to run from the resort but felt trapped. Planning travel in remote parts of India can be a logistical nightmare. I started tipping into a destructive headspace to escape in the only way I knew how. When B pulled out a bottle of vodka after everyone else had gone to bed, I drank a lot of it. I slept through the morning practice the following day and woke up to his face hovering over me. 'Drink this,' he said, shoving a fresh coconut in my hands, 'and don't tell anyone it was me.' He meant the vodka he had given me the previous night. Of course, he didn't force me to drink it, but he knew I was trying to stay away from alcohol and he had a duty of care.

Every day we would wake up, practise, and prowl around the resort like lions in captivity for the rest of the day then crawl back to our bedrooms. Amanda and I lay on our beds every night smoking hash that B had given us, which I had become an expert at shovelling into *beedis* (tobacco rolled in leaves) and plotting our escape. It wasn't easy because we were in the depths of Kerala, far from a train station, and the nearest village was an hour's walk away. We eventually managed to find a driver willing to get us into a nearby town and fled. B somehow found out where we went next and followed us. He gave up in the end but not without a lot of gaslighting and telling me that I was crazy because I had led him on. It took a long time to recover from that saga and I've been suspicious of gurus ever since – especially men. Wouldn't anyone be? I make no apology.

The Egomaniac

I once dropped into the class of a popular teacher in London to see what the hype was about. The first thing I noticed was that this man talked an awful lot. Fifteen minutes into the class and we hadn't started moving. *Just get on with the practice*, my mind screamed. Once we got to the postures, he walked around the room a little too fast in dizzying circles while giving us all a lecture on the meaning of yoga. I zoned inwards and focused on my breath. That is, until he started telling an anecdote from his travels, which involved doing the Indian accent of a guru he met in Calcutta. Everyone laughed. That was annoying but I was intrigued by this strange man whose class was full of people, most of whom seemed to be regulars. I kept moving and wondering what weirdness he might do next. His adjustments looked odd. He seemed to be doing a strange thing where he rubbed the base of the spine (to stimulate a chakra there?) when students were in Downward Facing Dog Pose. *How strange*, I thought, *please don't do that to me*. Thankfully I escaped that adjustment, but he came over to me when I was doing Navasana (Boat Pose) where you lean back with your legs in the air. It's a pose that's repeated five times in the Ashtanga sequence and in other drop-in classes sometimes up to three. We were all quite literally on our last legs. My belly was trembling, feet dropping towards my mat. I was about to give up when the teacher came over, grabbed my ankles and dragged me across to the front of my mat. Everyone started laughing again. I laughed too mostly because I couldn't believe what had just happened. I felt embarrassed. *What was the point of assisting like that?* I thought. Offering adjustments should be about love, guiding and showing the way or helping a person go deeper into a pose. I walked out of that class early.

It took several more years before I started refusing adjustments from teachers I didn't know. The first time was on holiday in Bali in 2018. I dropped into an Ashtanga class at a studio where the only Balinese people in the building appeared to be staff and everyone practising was travelling or newly settled in the gentrified neighbourhood with cafes that sold avocado on toast. I should have known then that this was probably not my kind of place.

The teacher grabbed my hips when I was doing a standing twist and I was so shocked I found myself saying 'I don't want to be adjusted, thank you,' before I could stop myself. Simple as that. It felt empowering to say no to a stranger but I was upset he hadn't asked. I know a lot of teaching involves a lot of trial (and hopefully less error) but I find it astounding when some dive in heavy-handedly, not knowing anything about the body (and emotional being living inside of it) they've set upon. I've never been in the business of assisting for the sake of it. I was taught not to do that, and I always ask. Assisting is about trust and forming a dialogue. It's also worth knowing how much you can help someone simply by pointing and talking too – you don't even have to touch them.

The Humiliator

I feel strongly about talking about abuse of power within yoga because it's not only high-profile cases that we need to be aware of. There are many other incidents going on under the radar. One such case led me to speak out – via a post on social media at first, which led to talks with the owners of a yoga studio but sadly nothing much changed. The story went like this.

Rachel (not her real name) was a newly qualified yoga teacher I met at one of the studios where I taught. I mentioned a teacher I had heard was difficult to work with. I didn't have any reasonable evidence for disliking him other than instinct; he had a creepy vibe and I'm smarter about listening to gut feelings these days. What I found most strange was that he had a huge following of mostly bendy acrobatic-looking women; from what I had seen, you would need that kind of body to get to the end of his class. It turned out that Rachel had her own story involving a run-in with this same teacher. She had been practising in his class when he instructed everyone to place their hand on their glutes while engaging those muscles at the same time. Rachel didn't want to. *Important sidenote: if you ever find yourself in a class where the teacher won't let you modify a pose to suit yourself – leave. It's your body, your choice.*

Unhappy with Rachel's disobedience, the teacher grabbed her hand and slapped it onto her bum with his hand on top, announcing something along the lines of 'This girl's so uptight she can't put her hand on her bum.' Rachel didn't complain to the studio because she was too busy crying after class and was worried that she was being oversensitive. She went home and told her girlfriend, who urged her to report the incident but Rachel didn't want to cause a fuss or rehash the trauma of the event again.

The next day I couldn't stop thinking about what Rachel had told me. How many other incidents like this have gone unnoticed? This thought kept whirring around my brain on a loop. *This can't happen again*, I thought, grabbing my phone. I wrote a social media post about what happened, careful not to identify Rachel or the teacher. I didn't ask Rachel's permission, which I should have done, but I was too angry to think things through. I was a relatively new teacher and had no reputation to protect by staying silent anyway. Coincidentally it was International Women's Day when I uploaded that post. I wasn't prepared for what happened next.

Messages started coming through almost immediately from yoga teachers. All of them said they knew who I was talking about, despite me not having revealed his name. These teachers with more experience and therefore more power than me knew and hadn't done anything. I felt deflated. One teacher who taught at the same studio told me stories of questionable behaviour that she had seen from this man before and expressed shame that she hadn't spoken up. She wanted to do so now by raising the incident with the studio's management. Screenshots of my post were shared with the studio owners and I was called in for a meeting. I wanted it all to go away by that point but this was a fiasco I had started and I was going to have to clear it up. I sent Rachel a text to tell her what I had done and luckily she didn't mind the story being public if it brought about change. She also agreed for me to include it in this book.

'Your social media's been causing a stir,' the owner of the studio where the offending teacher worked told me. I still wasn't sure what I had done wrong. He suggested Rachel make a formal complaint as otherwise there was little that the studio would be able to do. This annoyed me because he seemed reluctant to talk to the teacher, which seemed like the appropriate thing to do rather than pestering Rachel.

Several hours later, the studio owner sent me a text saying that they would be getting consent cards made to use in classes at the studio. These are cumbersome things that students can place on their mats if they don't want to be adjusted. I should have been proud of that moment. It was a small victory; I had brought about a tiny change – which is what Rachel had wanted – even if what I had done hadn't been formally acknowledged. A lot of yoga teachers stopped talking to me after that. At the same time, I saw social media posts popping up from teachers, some of whom had contacted me after my post, around the topic of consent and best practice for giving students adjustments. It wasn't long before consent cards started appearing for use in classes I taught myself. I didn't use them. If every teacher asked permission before offering adjustments, we wouldn't need them.

The teacher involved in this scenario was never publicly held accountable, but this has not been the case for other high-profile teachers. In 2012, John Friend, the founder of Anusara Yoga, admitted to sleeping with several students. He was also accused of running a Wiccan coven called Blazing Solar Flames, where members often went naked. In a public statement, Friend denied any involvement in 'a sex coven'. For a time he also withdrew from public life but has since launched another form of yoga, called Sridaiva.

Not all the recent scandals have been sexual; some have involved financial impropriety or the physical abuse of students. During his workshops, B.K.S. Iyengar, who died in Pune, India, in 2014, openly slapped and kicked his students while telling them 'It's not you I'm angry with, not you I kick.

It's the knee, the back, the mind that is not listening.' (from *The New Yorker*.)[14]

More recent, is the scandal I refer to as Ashtangate.

Ashtangate

Civil rights activist Tarana Burke began using the phrase Me Too in 2006 to raise awareness of women who had been abused. In 2017, it found global recognition amid allegations against Hollywood film producer Harvey Weinstein. Towards the end of the following year, yoga started having its own Me Too moment as news broke that Ashtanga guru Pattabhi Jois, who died in 2009 at the age of 93, had been a long-term abuser of students under his tutelage in Mysore. The first woman to speak out was Karen Rain. I remember scrolling through her blog when I first read her story, feeling sick but not shocked.

The allegations didn't affect me personally because, though I've practised Ashtanga yoga and visited Mysore, its birthplace, my introduction to the practice started with other teachers elsewhere. I was never taught by Pattabhi Jois myself and only met him briefly on that occasion when I roped my mum into making chai for him on his visit to London. I wasn't surprised by Rain's revelations because sexual assault in the yoga world wasn't new. According to the same 2019 article in *The New Yorker*,[15] more than a dozen former students have come forward to accuse Jois since 2010. Their allegations include that he rubbed his genitals against their pelvis while they were in extreme back bends, lay on top of them while they were prostrate on the floor, and inserted his fingers into their vaginas – an action that (and you won't believe this) fellow students excused as an adjustment to their mula bandha, believed to be the root lock or the body's lowest chakra, which lies at the pelvic floor.

The allegations threw the Ashtanga community worldwide into turmoil. Everyone was reeling. In some cases I saw yogis apparently justifying what Jois did by finding explanations or – in worst-case scenarios – blaming the victims. 'Was it possible to separate the man from the practice?' became a big question. *Well yes, of course*, I thought, *Jois didn't invent it*. Some senior teachers rightly spoke out against Jois, while lengthy social media posts and blogs started rolling out from people who had built careers attached to PJ's name. And yet, other famous teachers were incredulous and appeared to deny knowledge of the allegations, while others shamefully remained silent. It felt like I was witnessing an uncomfortable patriarchal spirituality that big yoga players were feeling forced to uphold because their own reputations were at stake.

Perhaps the hardest stories to digest were the confessions from yoga practitioners who admitted to knowledge of sexual abuse and didn't speak out at the time. Genny Wilkinson Priest, yoga manager at Triyoga, Europe's biggest group of yoga studios based in London, said as much in an article she penned for *Yoga Journal* in November 2018.[16] She writes: 'I'm ashamed to admit that I knew about the sexual assault soon after I first started a daily Ashtanga practice 17 years ago. While I practised with Jois several times before his death, I was not a close student of his and never saw the abuse first hand. But I did see videos on the Internet; I did laugh off and dismiss the furtive, dark gossip in Mysore, India, cafes and in practice rooms everywhere from New York to Singapore to London; and I did turn a blind eye.' On the ground, Ashtanga teacher friends of mine told me that, for reasons no one could explain, photos of Jois remained on the walls of studios where they practised. I couldn't understand why students didn't refuse to practise in these spaces until they were taken down. I also continued to see 'Practice and all is coming' – a famous quote of Jois' – on social media posts and chalked up on yoga studio blackboards for some time after the allegations were known. It was a good line, but I was confused about its continued use in light of what everyone now knew.

Another big question I had was when would Sharath, Jois' grandson and heir of the Ashtanga empire, say something? No one I asked seemed to know. The long-awaited and incredibly late-in-the-day statement from the K. Pattabhi Jois Ashtanga Yoga Institute eventually came in July 2019. In an Instagram post that has since been removed, Sharath Jois, current director of the Institute, acknowledged seeing his grandad sexually assault female yoga students who spoke out in 2018.

'It brings me immense pain that I also witnessed him giving improper adjustments,' Sharath wrote in the post. 'I am sorry it caused pain for any of his students. After all these years I still feel pain from my grandfather's actions.'

In a piece[17] on his website, yoga teacher and author Matthew Remski noted that the apology came more than a year after a feature piece[18] he wrote that presented the testimonies of nine women who alleged to have been abused by Jois. On his website, Remski, whose book *Practice and all is Coming*[19] centres the voices of some of Jois' victims and investigates the wider structural conditions that enabled such abuse, writes:

The context I'd like to provide here is with respect to the women who made Sharath's statement not only necessary, but possible, and whose names he does not mention.

Sharath's post comes nine years after the first published testimony by Anneke Lucas. It comes three years after a panel was convened in NYC at which Lucas was joined by another survivor; they both described Jois assaulting them. It comes a year and a half after Karen Rain's #metoo statement about Jois went viral and her activist writing on the issue started to take off.

Sharath's post led to 1,300[20] comments and other influencer teachers posting and blogging about the situation and finally offering their own apologies for not believing the women who spoke out too. One of them was Ashtanga megastar Kino MacGregor, who had upset victims in an initial statement, which Karen Rain responded to claiming that it appeared to minimize the assault allegations. In July 2019 in a blog on her own website MacGregor wrote a follow-up piece[21]:

At first I resisted the claims of sexual assault, calling the adjustments only inappropriate. I did not immediately side with the victims. Instead I searched for ways to justify the reported behavior, finding corroborating evidence in the testimony of students who said that they had in fact benefited from being touched in their genitalia by Jois. I have been slow to admit the faults of my teacher and quick to deflect and defend . . . A combination of loyalty and self-interest blinded me to reality. I'm sorry that it took me this long to see the truth.

Sharath's apology was 'liked' thousands of times.[22] I noted that the applause came mostly from Ashtanga heavyweights with giant followings, and big business. The apology was described as brave, though to me it lacked conviction. Some people said to give the guy a break, it's hard to speak up about sexual-related stuff in Indian culture. This is true; I understand how suppressed and taboo it can be to discuss sexual assault and anything relating to women's bodies. If the victims had been Indian women I doubt they would have spoken up for fear of being shamed, and there would have been no apologizing to do. As it was, many of Sharath Jois' customers are Westerners and they did speak up, and so it was only right that he put right what had gone wrong. Ultimately though, it didn't matter what the rest of us thought. I was only interested in what the victims – or perhaps it's better to call them survivors because that's what they have had to be – thought. Women like Karen Rain are the real heroes, and if anyone had been brave throughout the Ashtangate scandal it was no one else but them.

The allegations against Jois were just the latest in a string of scandals that date back decades. *The New Yorker*[23] reported:

> *In 1991, protesters accused Swami Satchidananda, the famous yogi who issued the invocation at Woodstock, of molesting his students, and carried signs outside a hotel where he was staying in Virginia that read Stop the Abuse. (Satchidananda denied all claims of misconduct.) In 1994, Amrit Desai, the founder of the Kripalu Centre for Yoga, a well-known yoga-retreat center, was accused of sleeping with his students while purporting to practice celibacy. (Desai eventually admitted to having sexual contact with three women.) More recently, Bikram Choudhury, the founder of 'hot,' or Bikram, yoga, has faced several civil lawsuits for sexual misconduct, including one filed in 2013 by his own lawyer, Minakshi Jafa-Bodden, who said that he not only harassed her but also forced her to cover up allegations of misconduct against other women. (Bikram has denied all allegations.)*

In 2019, Netflix released the documentary *Bikram: Yogi, Guru, Predator*, which I only managed to watch ten minutes of before I had to switch it off. I did return to finish watching the entire thing later and forced James to see it too so I didn't have to feel awful alone. 'Why are men so shit?' I asked him. James didn't have an answer and was sickened by the film too. As I stared at the documentary on my laptop screen, it boggled my mind how so many of Bikram's students spoke highly of him despite what he had been accused of. Others broke down in tears in the film in what looked like a combination of confusion, betrayal and disbelief. It's hard to believe that the man is still in business and people continue to flock to train with him.

I was keen to speak to one of my own Ashtanga teachers about the Pattabhi Jois scandal so I called Gingi from The Shala where I practised when it was in Clapham. Gingi co-founded The Shala, now in West Norwood, in 1997 with his wife Ella and it was the first dedicated Ashtanga studio established in London. He has been teaching yoga for more than twenty-five years (even longer than I have practised) and is one of the UK's most senior Ashtanga teachers. You wouldn't know it though, as he has hardly any public profile to speak of, which – going by today's standards, where online presence is social currency and a sign of moving up in the world – is a strange thing. Gingi's reputation speaks for itself among his students, many who have practised with him for a long time. I feel very lucky I met him when I did.

I asked Gingi what his impressions of Pattabhi Jois were since he had practised with him in Mysore.

I knew that there was something not quite right about him. He had a very strange relationship with money, and students would shower him in gifts. The rich students would bring him gold and if you didn't have any money he expected you to bring his coffee. There was also never any love in his adjustments and he seemed grumpy a lot of the time. He was friendly to some of the students but he wasn't very nice to me. I really wanted to feel the love for him because everyone else felt it. I spent a lot of time trying to work it out, trying to make him like me, and it never worked. I don't know whether he thought I had a big ego or what. I just didn't feel that he saw me.

'That's so sad,' I said, 'but also common in the yoga world these days where classes are sometimes huge and teachers don't always see you. That's what we all want, isn't it? To be acknowledged. I felt seen when I first came to The Shala. I really needed it back then.'

'It's so important, we all need that acknowledgement,' Gingi agreed. I asked Gingi if he was aware of sexual abuse going on at the time he was in Mysore.

I never saw anything happen, but there were a lot of rumours. We all just thought they couldn't be true. In hindsight I feel really upset about the fact that we chose not to believe the rumours, which is wrong.

I feel like I played a part in letting the abuse go on by refusing to see it. I also feel bad because I could have maybe done something. I should have listened to my instincts but I just kept my head down and focused on my practice. The Me Too movement helped me to speak up. I thought I was in the wrong when I knew something wasn't quite right so it's cathartic to talk about it now. I know lots of people were shocked because they've built their careers in Jois' name, but it offered an opportunity to reassess everything. I think a good question for us to think about in

light of everything we now know is whether Ashtanga is losing
something or is it gaining? I think seeing the practice for what
it is – beyond any guru – can be a good thing.

I couldn't agree more with Gingi. Of course, it's easier for me to separate Jois from my own experience of Ashtanga yoga because I didn't practise with him, but I think there's room for those who did to process and move through what has happened and for the practice itself to serve people as it always has.

Gingi grew up in San Francisco and had a martial arts background. His dad was a highly successful Sensei and taught in schools all over Europe where Gingi assisted him in the 1980s. At the age of nineteen he decided that path wasn't for him. 'I felt that I was always going to be in my father's shadow,' he told me, 'so I thought about what I might do instead. I moved to London and started exploring art school but soon I wasn't sure about that either. A few years later while travelling in India I discovered yoga for the first time. I met someone in Hampi who practised Ashtanga and we made a deal that he would teach me Ashtanga and I would teach him Tai Chi. I never ended up teaching him Tai Chi because I loved the yoga so much. I loved the flow of it, the strength and formality of it. I recognized the synchronicity and structure, which is central to martial arts so it was familiar to me. It just got me in a way I can't describe. Yoga found me. It was beautiful.'

Back in London, Gingi continued his practice with the late Derek Island, who he described as 'looking like a rock star'.

I remember seeing him through the window of the place that
he taught and thinking he doesn't look like a yoga teacher. He
was charismatic and charming and he flaunted himself a lot
but it was with a sense of fun. After being in India where yoga

seemed so serious, Derek taught it in a way that was with great
respect for the practice but we didn't take ourselves too seriously.
He wasn't trying to be some big guru either. I built The Shala
in his memory because he was ill for a long time and I found
a new place for him to teach because we thought he was going
to get better. But when he didn't I started teaching myself.

That sense of fun and playfulness in Derek is what I experienced through being taught by Gingi as well. This is how
I learnt that it's possible to be inspirational and have a noble
ethos, one that doesn't throw the ego out of check. Having a
kind and relatable teacher is what made Gingi fall in love
with yoga and has shaped both of our perceptions of the
practice and how we wanted to teach and be taught.

After several years of doing yoga classes as a punishing exercise because of the terrible relationship I had with my body,
Gingi taught me how to practise in a more compassionate way.
The Shala became a safe space for me to go to practise discipline
when everything else in my life felt out of control. And though
I've not practised regularly with Gingi for a long time because
I live further away, those early years had an impact. It was Gingi
who encouraged me to do a headstand, something I had avoided
for about ten years before, and he patted me on the back and
said 'it comes and goes' when I must have looked like I was
going to cry because a complicated posture I had mastered the
week before eluded me the next. He also told me to go further
in the Ashtanga Second Series (which I had been avoiding)
when I did an advanced teacher training course with him several
years ago. Gingi knew when to hold the space, and when to
gently push you. I've internalized these skills and they're part
of the way I practise and teach too. I think that's the mark of
a brilliant student–teacher relationship – one that I know he

has had with many others too. So I've always remembered the many often subtle things I learnt from Gingi. When I teach I like to push and encourage students too, but I try to do it in a way that means I'm there to support and be led by students so they don't go further than they're ready.

Given how pivotal my relationship with Gingi was in my own practice jorney, I wondered whether he thought the guru–student relationship could also be problematic. 'I think it's a big problem! I tried very hard never to be like that. Having a teacher to look up to is important but I shouldn't be your only teacher. I might have been practising longer than you, but I'm just here to show you the way. We're all equal – the practice teaches that – and ultimately we all have to find our own way. We're all evolving all the time – I am too. We shouldn't have a hierarchy.'

And does he think there is a way back for yoga like it was in his early days? 'I don't think so. It just seems to be getting bigger. It's a huge machine and it's so commercialized; I don't really understand it. I'm so glad we found yoga when it wasn't like this. I wouldn't know where to begin if I came to it now.'

I feel exactly the same. It's good to know I'm not alone, but I have to stay hopeful that things will change, that yoga commerce will fail and the machine might break down. The commercialized and commodified 'love and light' years of yoga have got to come to an end. The world needs something better.

CHAPTER 7

Endings, Beginnings

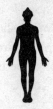

When I got back to London from that India trip with the bad guru in 2013 (see page 138), I gave up on yoga for a while. It was still several years before I started teaching yoga full-time and at that point I didn't think I ever would. Those months with that teacher in Kerala had destroyed yoga for me; I felt dirty and triggered with thoughts of his hands on my body every time I tried to practise. I was certain I was never going to let a man teach me again. I felt foolish and angry – with men but also with myself for thinking the trip would offer me salvation out of the booze-ravaged life I had been stuck in at the time. India, birthplace of yoga, had existed as a font of spiritual wisdom in my mind for so many years, and this now felt like a lie. I had invented a glossy narrative in my head when the reality had been a weird mess involving sexual harassment in public places and a teacher on a power trip. I may have had breaks from yoga in the past but this felt different, more final. There was no going back to the mat. Or so I thought.

I emailed Gingi to tell him what had happened: that India had been a waste of time and that I didn't think I could practise anymore. I wasn't sure what I would do to fill the inevitable spiritual void that would need filling but for now yoga and I were finished, I told him. Ironically in my complaints about gurus and yoga I was now looking to him to tell me what to do. Gingi advised that I shouldn't throw my practice away because of one bad experience. He also suggested that the trip may have been useful as a way of showing me how *not* to teach yoga if I ever wanted to teach in future. This made me feel better and helped me not to dismiss the trip as a waste of time, but it also clarified in my mind – at that point at least – that I didn't want to teach anyway.

If this book has felt like a big story of losing faith and finding it only to watch it slip away again, then that could be about right. Yoga has helped me out many times and sometimes it hasn't.

Giving Up, Starting Again

I'm going to take you back to 2017 when my grandmother died and a bit of me died too. I wasn't sure if I believed in anything anymore. All hope drained away. I know people for whom the death of a loved one has made their faith in life, their religion or practice stronger than ever. My mum's own faith was what kept her going through the same loss. This wasn't how it went for me, which leads me to question how strong my practice might have been in the first place. Maybe it wasn't very strong or my practice hadn't been put to the test yet.

Although I've talked a bit about my experiences of teaching yoga already, at that time I still hadn't started doing it full-time. Teaching yoga, something I hadn't seriously considered before became my way of dealing with grief. In this way, my grandmother's death led to one of the most significant rebirths of my life, which has changed its trajectory in recent years. 'Life changes fast. Life changes in the instant.' the writer Joan Didion tells us in her memoir[24] about her husband's death, and that's how it went for me. I moved through the early months following my grandmother's death feeling as if my limbs had been blown off. There was a giant hole in my stomach that felt like it would never heal. The emptiness was so vast there was no room to let any other feelings in. I no longer had a way to fill that hole because I didn't drink anymore. I wondered again about the meaning (if any) of life. *What's the point of it all?* became a nagging thought that hovered over my head like a giant question mark. It's at moments like that, when life feels razed to the ground, that there's nothing left to do but stay where you are surrounded by the rubble until you've got the strength to build it back up. We buried my nan on New Year's Eve. My family and I had spent over a week in hospital with her, waiting for this moment and yet it was still surreal watching her stiff body disappear down a hole. My brain couldn't compute what I was witnessing. *I will never see her again,* I told myself as bearded men shovelled moist soil over the top. I watched my mum scatter rose petals over her grave. 'You had better live to be a hundred,' I whispered to her.

'I intend to, *Inshallah,*' she said and we both smiled sadly, tears spilling down our faces. I scooped up a handful of petals and shoved them into my coat pocket, trying to keep a piece of my grandmother with me.

* * *

My nan had been such a formidable woman that I thought she would outlive us all. It was both a slow and sudden death. Slow because she was in hospital for over a week and abrupt because I was standing outside a yoga studio about to drop off a Christmas present for a teacher friend when the texts came through. It was another stroke, they said; she was unlikely to come home. *Life changes fast. Life changes in the instant.* I didn't understand. My nan was made of steel, she'd had several strokes, urinary tract infections, diabetes and high blood pressure, and had always pulled through. The next day I travelled up to the hospital in Oxford, still not convinced it was happening. But there she was, surrounded by her children. It was true. It could be days, weeks, but it would happen.

We set her up with headphones and a man with a beautiful voice reciting the Quran in her right ear without knowing for sure if she could hear. Prayers were performed around her bed and everyone said what they needed to. I whispered that I loved her and left it there. Ours was an uncomplicated relationship with no history to repair.

No one knew her real birthday, but the hospital wrist-band said 8 March 1938. That's what had gone on the immigration papers. It was clearly entirely coincidental, but I love the fact that it's the date for International Women's Day. Because what a woman she was. She was widowed at thirty-five, with six children aged sixteen to three, in London, which was still a foreign city for her. Then fifteen years later, one of her daughters was killed in a car crash at the age of twenty-one. My nan never recovered. How can you?

An ambulance had taken her to the hospital four days before Christmas. A fortnight earlier I had spent a week caring for her. She hadn't been unwell but was frail and not as mobile as she had been in former years. I practised handstands against a wall as she watched, lying on her side in bed and smiling at me. We laughed as I struggled to drag her higher onto the pillows so she could see me properly. As I heaved and puffed,

I remember thinking this wasn't a great existence for a woman who had been so active. I plaited her hair, lit her cigarettes and got her to tell me – again – about living in Lahore after she was married, because it made her face light up.

Men don't feature heavily in my formative years. I come from a matriarchal lineage of strong women. Strong not because they were made that way but because they had to be, and it was my grandmother who had paved the way. She had been a force of nature and, alongside my mum, is one of my biggest inspirations. I adored her and called her Biggie as a child because she was adamant she was too young to be a grandma, aged forty-two when I was born. She wanted to be Big Mum to my real mum which was fitting because she had been a second parent to me in the absence of my dad. She always had a hundred things to do and was permanently on her way somewhere – running errands, taking English lessons or aqua aerobics classes. Nothing got in the way of doing what she set out to do so she often took me with her. When my mum was at work, Biggie would be in the playground wearing salwar kameez and trainers to pick me up after school. She did that for almost a year before the other kids and teachers realized she wasn't my actual mum.

She had a tough life as a single mother, working long hours as a machinist in a factory for high-street fashion outlets. She would take extra work to do at home, where there were always bundles of clothes, loose threads, piles of zips everywhere. She had also been a hard woman to love sometimes. She was depressed after her daughter died, had what appeared to be an acute, but sometimes dormant, form of schizophrenia. It can be a scary mental illness – and is not one many people want to talk about. It's the kind of illness that makes people frightened of you so that they cross the road to avoid you or switch seats on the bus. But Biggie had never lashed out at me as she sometimes did to her children. It was like I wasn't in the room or didn't pose a threat. I got used to watching her in utter confusion when she was hearing voices and to hearing her ranting at them, and I would wait for her to go back to being the Biggie I knew and loved.

As I watched her dying, passing away, disintegrating, I saw what looked like the mental illness leaving her face. Witnessing her death approach felt like a privilege, but an invasion of her privacy. I was seeing her at her most vulnerable. *Please don't die*, I thought at the same time as thinking *will you hurry up if it makes the pain go away?* As the days went on, her masks fell off entirely, there was no pretending, no holding things together or putting a brave face on. She was letting life go and serenity seemed to be taking its place. Biggie had had a huge impact on my life and taught me many things. Here she was teaching me how to die. I wondered whether this is what she had wanted years ago when her daughter was killed but she'd had to carry on for the rest of us. When life's hard we have to keep going for other people, like John had told me all those years ago.

I was inconsolable watching her wilt and change colour while pretending to keep it together. Her skin turned pallid, almost golden and yet she was becoming more beautiful than I had seen her in years. People often talk about loved ones who have died as 'gone', but as the days went on I believed she had already gone. What makes a person who they are but their energy, their eyes, their smile? None of that was there anymore. Her body was breathing, but it was also decomposing, her brain closing down. It was like being confronted with the cruel reality of Savanana (Corpse Pose) and what that posture means in terms of the unification of mind and body. In the end, there's no mind, no body, just consciousness. And yet I was clinging onto her body, a metaphor for a life that once was. Doctors came into the room we had taken over and said 'She's not in any pain,' and I would wonder how they could possibly know. The room where it all happened: prayers, takeaways, sleepless nights on foam cushions laid out on the floor. Conversations, memories, jokes about how annoying and blunt Biggie could be, but also how funny and kind too. I spent a lot of those days walking around the hospital, eyeing up smokers in the car park and weighing up whether it could be justified if I relapsed into drinking or buying some tobacco. Christmas Day came, we pulled crackers over nut loaves in an otherwise empty hospital canteen. We shared memories of past Christmases with Biggie, ignoring the unbearable fact that there wouldn't be any more like them again.

Her death took ten days and we'll never know why. As her body shut down, her heart appeared to beat stronger than before. Then one day it stopped. It happened when there were only three of us in the room; my mum (her eldest child), my aunt (her youngest) and I (her first grandchild) were sitting around the bed. *Had she known?* I wondered. *Had it been her plan all along to slip away without a fanfare when everyone else was out of the room?* It was awful that she was dead, but it was also a relief. We couldn't wait anymore. I was holding her hand when she gurgled out her last hoarse breath. The three of us looked at each other. None of us could believe it. *Is this what death is?* I thought. *One breath in and they're here, another breath out and they're gone.* It didn't feel real. I snatched my hand away. This was it. This was actually it. There's nothing more raw or that makes you more sharply aware of being alive, than staring death in the face. Nothing. I walked out of the room not knowing where to go but I didn't know what else to do. I ran down the corridor and out into the car park, dreading what would happen next. I thought about asking a stranger for a cigarette but knew there was no point. I sat on the kerb, hugging my knees and waited when there was no more waiting to do. She was dead. She was dead. She was dead.

My mum was still sitting by the bed when I went back inside. I looked at the body, looked at my feet and looked at the body again, hoping a doctor would come in and tell us it had been a false alarm. But no, several staff arrived, wrapped her body in white sheets and slid it onto a trolley resembling a large incubator. My mum and I walked behind as they wheeled it out to a lift. I kissed her forehead when I saw the body at the mosque for the funeral the next day but I didn't know why. I felt suddenly detached, estranged and aware of the attachments we make to bodies of those we love, to our own. Sitting next to Biggie's body wasn't a comfort because I knew she wasn't there. And it made me question my attachments to my own body, the obsessiveness of those years when I starved and made myself sick, tried to control this body and distort it into something different. I felt foolish. We are not our bodies; bodies don't matter, I told myself as I sat cross-legged on the floor with a shawl on my head.

In the weeks and months that followed, my mind was constantly sifting through memories, looking for old pictures of the past and clinging onto them when I found them. I couldn't walk past a Boots store without going in to spray myself with Biggie's smell: Chanel No.5. I wallowed in memories of wet kisses, her touching my face or squashing a £20 note from her pension into my hand. I went further back to my childhood and remembered her putting henna on my hands using a matchstick because I loved it, and rubbing jasmine oil in my hair in the vigorous way Pakistani elders do. 'The people you love become ghosts inside of you and like this you keep them alive,' poet and artist Robert Montgomery known for his installations in public places tells us. I never wanted Biggie's ghost to leave. I saw her in my mum's face and I saw my mum's hands in mine. If I think carefully, I can remember the feel of Biggie's clammy palms when I held her warm hand, crêpe-paper skin, soft. That's the kind of ghostly memory I want to keep alive.

There was no room for yoga in my life after Biggie died. My mum tried to push me back towards it, knowing that it had helped when I'd returned to it in the past. I couldn't. I didn't want to process the grief, which I knew that yoga would require me to do. But when people have asked me why I started teaching yoga, it's obvious. When someone close to you dies, you find out very fast that life will never be the same. You don't want it to be.

'Why don't you try the gym?' was James's gentle attempt to nudge me towards doing something – anything – that might make me feel better. I had been dragging myself in to a communications job at a crowdfunding platform, unable to find any enthusiasm for anything, not in working, not in living. My manager eventually suggested I take gardening leave until I worked out whether I wanted to stay. I wasn't exactly sacked, but it felt like that might be coming. I called my boss after a fortnight to tell him I wasn't coming back. I put the phone down and sat on my bed in Peckham where I lived at the time, wondering what I was going to do with my life now. My mum told me to take some time out, which I did for a month, but nothing changed. James and I had only been together for a year up to that point. He had been doing all the right things to comfort me. Coming over at the last minute to stay the night when I asked (we didn't live together), preparing dinner or going to get a spliff off a friend when I told him it might help me sleep. He didn't complain when I pushed him away or cancelled dates we had planned because I couldn't get out of bed. He could see the longer I stayed away from yoga the worse things might get for me. He also knew that the biggest shifts in my life have happened when I've taken drastic action to shake myself up, and that's why he suggested I join the gym. It didn't immediately appeal. I was scared of gyms. I've felt feeble and incompetent every time I have found myself in one. The clank of machines, buff bodies, and mirrors were intimidating. But my view was about to change. I joined the local leisure centre and converted overnight. I didn't always enjoy being in yoga studios because of the lack of diversity among the usual clientele, but at the leisure centre I felt comfortable and blended in.

Lifting weights was near impossible for my trembling arms at first. I didn't know what a deadlift or a clean and press was when I arrived. I stood in the middle of a sports hall like the one in the YMCA where I went to my first yoga class, holding a barbell and was completely confused by the words coming out of the fitness instructor's mouth. My heart began pounding from the unexpected exertion within minutes of the warm-up, sweat soiled my T-shirt almost immediately and I felt like I might pass out several times. An hour later and I was buzzing. I suddenly wanted to feel strong again; I was determined and this could be the ticket to get there. I bounced out to the main gym, where James was doing bench presses (I know what those are now).

'THAT WAS A-MAZ-ING!' I shouted into his happy-looking face. The gym became an obsession. Not for weight-loss but for its own sake. I became hooked on feeling strong, and weights, circuits and barbells were what did it for me now. I went to classes every day for several months and it wasn't long before I was getting on my yoga mat again at home, which is always a sign that life is going as it should.

As part of my new regime, I dropped into a yoga class to see what it was about. I was blown away by how diverse it was. The teacher was a Black woman and everyone else looked like the people I saw outside in the neighbourhood too. It was a mixed bag of ages, skin colours, languages spoken. I felt at home. Leisure centres, like libraries (sadly rare these days), are one of my favourite places. If you want a snapshot of what a diverse community looks like, you won't find it in your local yoga studio – it's in your leisure centre, so go there. Diversity aside, I had come across some snobbery about yoga teaching in gyms. I'm not sure why. It could be because the level of qualification needed isn't the same as a yoga studio might demand. It feels that part of the hype around yoga these days is that it needs to be learnt through a specialist training body (with a premium price tag). But when we live in a yoga world filled with crash courses in how to teach, I'm not sure there's much difference.

Given my preoccupation with weights, the yoga class itself felt dull; I didn't like the sequence and it didn't push me enough. The teacher also made some ill-advised comments: 'You're moving too fast,' she told a speedy yogi in the front row. 'I'm the teacher so don't move on to the next pose until I say.' But it's thanks to her class that I had an epiphany. Lying there in Savasana, a pose designed for meditation and deep relaxation, my mind danced around with thoughts.

I could do this.

I want to do this.

And doing it in a leisure centre is exactly where I should start.

I left that class feeling renewed. I went home and cobbled together a yoga CV, compiling every scrap of yoga-related workshop and training I had ever done, and trawled online looking for jobs. I didn't get very far because jobs such as this aren't generally advertised. But I was determined and started emailing yoga studios directly. Most of them didn't respond, while others suggested I take classes at their studios to get a foot in the door (who has time to do that when you already have your own practice and teachers to guide you in place?). Most of them told me to try again when I had two years' teaching experience. It was true that I lacked experience, but the reasons why didn't always make sense. One of the best rejection letters I got went like this: 'Thanks so much for sending through your CV. I'm afraid we require more city studio experience to teach at our studios. But many thanks for your interest!' Which got me wondering what does city studio experience even mean? Another studio owner told me she was 'looking for cover teachers with a strong dynamic approach to Vinyasa Flow and Mandala' but she would keep me in mind if something came up. Again I was confused, thinking but what is Ashtanga if not a strong dynamic approach?

My lack of experience was what led to me volunteering with the charity that ran classes for refugees and asylum seekers. I still wasn't 100 per cent sure why I felt so persistent about pursuing yoga teaching without giving it much thought. I hadn't planned to teach, but I hadn't planned much in my life so far, I reasoned with myself. Why not give it a go?

After losing all faith when Biggie died, this was the first flicker of hope I had felt in months. It was making me feel human again so I was convinced it *had* to be my way forward. The first thing that had given my life meaning as a troubled teenager was yoga, and my favourite part of my teacher training in

London years later had been thinking about yoga all day. It made sense that I felt being immersed in the practice and filling my life with everything to do with it would bring me the peace and direction I needed. But too much of a good thing can go wrong very quickly, as I was soon to find out.

CHAPTER 8

Nice Work if You Can Get It

I was lucky enough to get the first yoga teaching job I auditioned for, at the UK's largest provider of leisure centres. Auditions (more on them later) are the yoga world's version of an interview. It wasn't for a permanent role, but it meant I was approved to be a substitute teacher at venues all over London. The first public class I taught in this job was at a leisure centre near the Arsenal football stadium in North London. The Ashtanga class was scheduled for mid-morning on a Sunday and I was so nervous I arrived forty-five minutes too early. I wandered the grounds, smiling at everyone I saw just in case they came to the class. I sat on some grass near the centre's tennis courts watching men with strong arms play. Time was moving so slowly I decided to go and have a look at the studio where I would be teaching, thinking it might calm my nerves.

No such luck. The studio door was bolted shut so I sat on the floor outside and waited, trying to take deep breaths and eat an apple at the same time. Minutes later, dozens of people started arriving and queuing outside. They seemed to be regulars, greeting each other, catching up, comfortable in their skins, happy to be here. I tried not to stare from where I was still on the floor, cramming the last bites of my apple, stressing myself out about what I had got myself into.

They don't know it's me taking the class, I thought.

Probably because I don't look like a yoga teacher.

Will they know it's my first time?

I don't want to do this anymore . . .

Oh shit. Too late.

The door was flung open and sweaty bodies started walking out. Then everyone outside started piling into the room. I followed them inside in a dreamlike daze and watched everyone confidently collecting mats, choosing their props and finding a spot to practise. *Oh man, this is really happening,* I thought, *and no one knows it's me taking the class.* My stomach tightened. I picked up a mat and walked to the front of the room, inhaling deep breaths in, long breaths out as best as I could. My mind was still struggling to catch up with my body. I watched my hands laying down the mat but they didn't look like they belonged to me. *Was I even really here?* I thought.

I eventually turned around to introduce myself to ALL THIRTY-ONE OF THEM. I had never talked to a room filled with so many people, all looking at me, awaiting instruction. I was going to be here for ninety minutes. No one seemed disappointed that I was standing in for their usual teacher as I had expected, which helped me feel slightly better about being there. Of course I didn't tell them it was my first time. I asked everyone to find a seated position they liked and to close their eyes if they felt comfortable in order to buy some time and guided them through an arrival, setting up an awareness of body and breath to get started.

My voice shook for the first fifteen minutes as we moved through Sun Salutations and most of the standing poses of the sequence. But as I walked around, assisting people with their postures, something shifted for me. I became so deeply absorbed in what we were doing together and aware that this is what teaching was meant to be. My focus was meant to be on the people in the class, but I'd lost sight of that because I'd been so caught up in my own fears. The class was about them – not me. The more I kept my attention on the people in front of me, the easier it felt. I became comfortable and the process started to flow. I kept walking around the room so that I could see everyone and they could see me.

I love offering students adjustments unless anyone has said they don't want to be assisted (and I always encourage people to say no if they want to). For many people, being helped by your teacher is one of the perks of going to a class. It is for me too, but only when I know and trust the teacher. I think too many newer teachers adjust for the sake of it. I've been assisted badly and didn't find it helpful. Learning adjustments was my favourite part of my teacher training and the first thing about teaching that I felt most confident with. I'm never heavy-handed when I meet a new group but that's another reason I walk around so much. You can gather a lot of data about people's bodies by watching them move through a series of yoga postures and make judgement calls on how you might help them. Sometimes I might just offer gentle hands-on-the-back, to let people know I've seen them. I felt conscious of this when I started teaching because I've been to so many classes where I've felt invisible. I never wanted to be that kind of teacher. Sometimes the reassurance of a hand on the back alone can help people go deeper into a posture – without me doing much at all. This is also a way of saying that I care, and a sort of 'well done' for getting on their mat because I know how hard it can be sometimes. As the class came to an end, I was exhausted but also anxious or maybe excited at the same time. I couldn't believe what I had just done. I thanked everyone for having me, walked over to a large window and stuck my head out of it, hoping they would all leave quickly just in case I burst into tears. I had no detailed memory of the class. Had it gone well? Could I do all of that again? I had no idea. A man came over and said, 'That was great. I've never done some of those poses before.' I had helped him get into his first head-stand. A woman mentioned that she loved my voice, which both surprised and pleased me because I'm often self-conscious of how deep it is. Another woman said she liked an adjustment I'd given her while she was doing a spinal twist. Others asked if I had any permanent classes at the centre and were disappointed when I told them I didn't. I felt overwhelmed. What wonderful people they were to take the time to connect with me. I felt excited, happy and hyper. I felt accepted. I'll always remember that first class and am deeply grateful to those who came. They didn't know it, but they were part of a huge milestone for me and I couldn't have asked for a more confidence-boosting first experience. But it didn't last long, because I had to keep looking for work, and that meant going to more auditions.

Auditions Aren't Just for Actors

Auditions are bizarre. Every single one I've done wasn't for an actual job but to go on the books to cover for resident teachers like I did at my first class. What happens is that you go along and teach a sequence of about ten minutes to other people also going for the same job while gym bosses and studio owners watch. The whole audition usually lasts for two hours, so it was hard not to feel inconvenienced. I understood the need for a process, but I was given the first three weekly classes

I later ended up teaching by meeting the owners of yoga studios for a chat, which felt like a more effective approach than watching a conveyor belt of people rattling through a tiny routine. Some places asked you to teach an unpaid one-hour class instead, which felt worse initially and ethically wrong, but I did it anyway.

It took a week of angst to prepare for my first audition for the job that led to that class I taught in North London. As soon as I arrived, I hid in the loo, texting James, who said: 'Breathe deep as I guess you already are,' which was useful because I wasn't. Having calmed down a little, I didn't know where to go, so sat on a leg press machine in the gym, hoping someone would look for me.

I couldn't have asked for a better first experience. The head of fitness who met me was an absolute joy: a Black man, gay, who was the same sort of age as me and had grown up in East London – also same as me. It was like seeing parts of myself reflected back. He ushered me into a huge airy studio, which sent my heart racing again – big rooms had that effect on me. Thankfully he batted away the part of the audition that involved watching me teach, which was a relief despite all the preparation I had done, and we ended up just having a chat. He was impressed with how long I had stuck with yoga through my life and had no interest in my lack of teaching experience, which was another reason I warmed to him more. Instead he asked me lots of probing questions about what I thought made a great yoga teacher, and how I would deal with tricky and emergency scenarios, which I appreciated. It felt nice to be grilled on the reasons I wanted the job. It made me feel valued and taken seriously.

I got the job and started covering classes at leisure centres all over London almost immediately. All of the classes I taught were in huge rooms that usually filled up with a mix of people, so I got lots of practice to help me get over my fear of facing large rooms and overcoming my anxiety around public speaking. I was intrigued by the range of those who came to class: people of colour, men, women, young, old, people with injuries or disabilities. I've rarely seen this happen in two decades of attending classes in London myself. Even in India, where I've done loads of yoga, the classes were exclusively taught by Indian men and participants were able-bodied or bendy tourists and the only other person close to being Indian in the room was me. From what I saw, leisure centres seemed to better reflect the communities that they were based within. It could simply be down to affordable pricing, the range of activities on offer, or because people feel comfortable in them (as I do because it feels that anyone and everyone is welcome).

My second audition was for a high-end gym chain at a branch in West London. It took me almost two hours on three trains to get there from where I lived in South London. I knew I wouldn't be able to do that journey regularly and I felt stupid for not having thought this through before. I walked into the building not sure I wanted the job anymore but decided that I needed to practise my public speaking so it could be a worthwhile thing to see through. The mind-and-body studio tucked at the end of a long corridor was predictably pretty, with a parquet floor and leaf-print walls. Everyone – all women bar one man who had the physique of a bodybuilder – was wearing their yogic best. We're talking Om tattoos, henna hands, Indian deities on tops. I looked like an extension of the wallpaper, wearing what later became my uniform: a pair of multicoloured flower-print leggings that I was convinced made me look like a yoga teacher from the pictures I had seen of yogis on social media, and a black top to quieten my bottom half down.

The staff at that audition weren't the friendliest. A young man with hard biceps and curvy calf muscles told us that there were twenty people to get through and only one job. 'The bar is higher here than at other places so we will be expecting you all to work hard to impress us,' he told us. *Crikey,* I thought, *should I just leave now?* Then he looked at me and said, 'Do you want to go first?' I kept things simple, set the scene by getting everyone in a seated position, and asking them to become aware of their bodies, their breathing and then led them through a few Sun Salutation As and Bs. I had an idea of how I felt yoga should be presented in gyms – in an accessible way. I do refer to yoga philosophy and remind people why we might be doing this practice but if you're teaching people who only come to class once a week, piling on the Sanskrit and bucketloads of chanting, which some of the others did, still doesn't feel right to me.

The hench bodybuilder bloke got up to audition next, wearing a tight vest paired with what I can only describe as tiny gym briefs (they looked like underwear) and five-finger barefoot shoes. He grabbed a pile of yoga blocks and started throwing them out at each of us. 'We're not going to be doing any Om-ing or New Age chanting,' he told us. *I'm sorry what? New Age?* I looked at the woman on the mat next to me, who sighed and raised her eyebrows back. Everyone looked confused. Mr Barefoot then proceeded to teach the strangest yoga I've possibly ever experienced. At one point we were trying to balance one foot on two blocks with the other still on the floor, doing yoga poses that were vaguely familiar but frankly felt wobbly and stressful.

'It's all very well trying to be flexible,' he said but this thing he was showing us was going to make us strong. *I'd rather be lifting weights to achieve that,* I thought as I tried to cross one leg over the other into an Eagle Pose while still wobbling around on the blocks. I found out later that he had received investment for this yoga block idea on an entrepreneurial TV show so there was clearly interest in the method even if he hadn't managed to convince anyone in the room that day. Two of the other candidates were kind enough to tell me that they enjoyed my piece as we collected our coats to leave, but I didn't get the job.

I was called for an interview by the owner of an art gallery who planned to open a wellness studio in the building's basement. I clocked that there were no windows as she showed me around and, in the event of an emergency, no obvious quick exits. My mind started wandering off on worst-case scenarios. What if there was a fire upstairs while we were blissfully meditating under blankets downstairs? Would anyone remember to save us? The owner looked at me expectantly, so I launched into my *Here's what I'm about* speech. Halfway through I got the sense she wasn't really getting it. 'I'm not sure what style of yoga you prefer,' I said, expecting her to fill me in. But no, it turned out she had never practised yoga before but was launching this new business because 'yoga's really trendy at the moment, isn't it?'

It's at meetings like that where you realize you're interviewing your prospective employer as much as they are you. I knew then that this arrangement wasn't going to work for me. But just in case I needed confirmation, I asked how the business model would work. She told me that she would offer the studio as an empty space for yoga teachers to hire and bring in their own students. All payments would be split 60:40 in her favour. I walked out not sure what to do. I was still at the start of my teaching journey, had no business flair or any clue how to start promoting myself. I wanted life to be simple and to be able to just walk in, take a class and get paid, so I said no to that one.

I interviewed for another leisure centre provider that was twenty minutes from where I lived. The wages were pitiful at £25 per class but the prospect of work so close to home enticed me. I turned up dressed, rehearsed and ready for the part, but there had been an internal communications breakdown and they'd forgotten about me. The duty manager was fetched, and we sat on chairs by the entrance for a hurried fifteen-minute conversation. She admitted that she hadn't looked at my CV and didn't know anything about yoga so I felt like a bit of an idiot talking about it. She then made a phone call to her mum halfway through my beginner's guide to yoga to arrange for her kids to be picked up from school, so things weren't going well. I didn't hear anything for a month and when I followed up, I received an automated email that said: 'Other candidates matched the profile we were looking for more closely.' So that was that.

I auditioned at an Essex branch of the gym that I had been to in West London. Given the whole 'bar is higher' scenario from last time, I was reluctant to go but my mum convinced me that it would be good practice. There were only four of us this time and the whole experience felt more comprehensive. The head of fitness was warm and friendly. She explained how things worked for freelancers on the payroll and even took part in the audition, which I thought was a nice touch. Several days later she got in touch full of compliments with an offer to teach a weekly Ashtanga class. I really wanted to take it because I liked her but turned it down because the travel costs and time wouldn't have made it worth it. The more fascinating point was the soap opera behind the class's availability. The existing Ashtanga instructor had been sacked the previous night when a Zumba class in an adjoining studio had run ten minutes over when the Ashtanga class started.

The yoga teacher had stormed into the Zumba class, shouting 'keep the fucking noise down' in front of everyone. True story.

The weirdest part of my job-seeking adventure didn't even involve an audition. I'd pinged off my CV to a bunch of studios, asking them to get in touch if they had work. I was indiscriminate in the early days and emailed almost every studio in London (although never up west again; I had learnt my lesson). Twenty minutes later I was on a bus to the gym for my barbell fix when an email came through from a woman saying she had two 7 a.m. classes that paid £20 each and asking if she could put me down to start next week. This was a bit hasty, even for a speedy person like me. The pay was low too but as I was starting out, I thought I should probably go for it. I thought it over while on the treadmill and decided that I should slow things down a bit. I emailed back asking if I could have some time to work out my availability. She somehow took that as me accepting her offer, sent me a document including an access code to get into the building, instructions for how to register students and details on how I'd be fined £20 on occasions I didn't find cover for classes I couldn't take. I was confused. I looked the woman up online and discovered the studio had been featured in a national news piece three days earlier. I didn't like the sound of it but, just in case I was wrong, I texted Melanie to ask what she thought. Was I being a fool to turn away an opportunity even though the pay was so low and the woman was willing to employ me without us having met? Mel advised that I arrange a meeting before taking on any work. But by the time I got home I received another email from the studio owner saying I was on the class timetable with classes starting the following week. I checked the website and there I was; she'd found a (terrible) headshot of me on the internet. It was too weird.

I emailed and said I didn't think we were the right fit for each other. She got back and said she was confused. I ghosted her. I had no choice.

As a laugh I emailed what's been reported as one of the most expensive gyms in the world and was surprised when I was invited to join an audition. The week before the scheduled audition I received a follow-up email saying that the group of applicants had grown bigger so could we do five minutes of teaching instead of the usual ten? *No problem*, I thought. *We can fit three Sun Salutations into that time.* It wasn't to be. The day before the audition, I got another email asking for three minutes of our 'best material'. Material?

'This is yoga we're talking about, not stand-up comedy,' I yelled at my phone. 'What the hell do they expect me to do in three minutes, for fuck's sake?' I asked James. 'How can they even make a decision on someone in that time?'

I wasn't sure I could be bothered to trek to St James's Park for this nonsense. I texted a friend who was better at staying calm than me to check if I was being too hot-headed in turning it down. He replied: 'Hit them with your serious punk, recoverist yang spiel, then do a mind-blowing break-dancing Sun Salutation and drop the mic.' I decided not to go. I emailed the gym back, explaining that I was teaching in Covent Garden earlier (which was true) and wouldn't make it in time (a lie). The organizer, who I must admit was very polite, emailed me back saying that she had checked Google Maps and I should still be able to make it after my class.

Urgh. This is why lying is bad. So I sent her this:

Apologies – it's a 90 min class I'm teaching so I think it'll be a bit rushed to make it for a three min audition. Sad to miss out, though not sure what impression I'd be able to make in that time.

Ending on a point of honesty made my soul feel a bit cleansed after all those lies.

For all the tragic-comedy of these auditions, I hated attending them but they were necessary. One of the more brutal ones was at a growing company whose representative described it as the 'Starbucks of Yoga' on account of the speedy rate at which it had opened multiple studios. It was a warm Saturday afternoon. The recruiter, Fi, arrived twenty minutes late, while the other candidates and I waited outside, pretending to be interested in meeting one another. I was the only person of colour as usual and no one else had been to an audition before. I wasn't in the mood to explain the ropes or make new friends and so sat on the pavement, gazing into the middle distance until we were let in.

Fi had long balayage dyed hair, wrists jangling with beads and threaded bracelets and several Sanskrit tattoos. Most prominent was one of the Om symbol, which always sinks my heart.

Om (pronounced *Ah*, *Oh*, *Mm*) is considered the most sacred mantra in Hinduism and Tibetan Buddhism. It appears at the beginning and end of most Sanskrit chants and prayers. Om is believed to contain the entire universe. It's a vibration from which the universe emanates. It's the first sound babies make when they're born and the last sound we make when we die. Isn't that just amazing? Think about it for a moment. All humans make a version of Om with our mouths – going from parted lips (*Ah* and *Oh*) to closed (*Mm*) – in both birth and death, whether we emit a sound or not. Om contains the past, the present, and the future: all that was, all that is, all that will be. In some ways, it could be the sound of a powerful void. I once dropped into a class where the teacher, who had a huge social media following, declared: 'Om means "YES".' I was disappointed. It's bigger than that. Its symbol is also believed to be sacred, and thus probably not something to parade casually on your arm, unless you deeply understand its meaning.

Fi told us she'd started yoga six years earlier and then left a finance job to become a teacher. She also confessed that she was hungover. We candidates each took turns to teach for ten minutes, while Fi made notes on her iPhone. I taught some standing poses from the Ashtanga Primary Series but she cut me off when I had everyone standing on one leg, saying she'd seen enough.

'Are you Ashtanga trained?' Fi asked. I looked at her and nodded, assuming that she was talking to me, because it was obvious from what I'd taught. But she was looking at someone else who'd delivered a generic series of flowing movements that could have been described as several different styles of yoga. It was becoming clear who her favourites were. Was I deluding myself with this job-hunting? I felt despondent about being critiqued by someone who seemed to epitomize 'the look' of what a yoga teacher was meant to be, which was something I'd never acquire. Was it because I wasn't jazzy or funky enough? Maybe the postures I taught weren't fun enough, or perhaps it was because I didn't have enough 'good vibes'. I suddenly felt like an outlier within yoga, the very thing that had so often kept me going in my life.

Afterwards, I got on the train to go home, feeling wiped out and with several emotions rising in me that I couldn't name. Anger, sadness, tension, fed up? I didn't know. As I got closer to home in South-east London, I started shaking, not visibly, but on the inside. At each station the train filled with more people. I became breathless like I was going to explode. I felt drowsy and started to see black spots around other passengers' faces. I stared at shoes, brogues, ballet pumps, those awful boat shoes men wear without socks. Converse, Nike, Vans. I made it to my stop and, once home, sat immobile on the sofa. My phone rang; it was my mum. It wasn't long before I started crying. Hearing my mum's voice does that to me when I'm upset. I relayed what had happened at the audition.

'Maybe you should stop the auditions for a while if they're making you anxious,' my mum said. 'But it's the only way I can get work,' I told her. She replied: 'I don't think it's worth it, Nadi. Focus on your own practice. That's the most important thing for you.' It was sound advice and the truth.

Several days later when I was calmer, I followed up with Fi who told me that she hadn't seen enough of me, and could I send her a video of myself teaching? She hadn't 'seen' me because she hadn't looked closely. And who has videos of themselves teaching? Everything about that audition – the judgement, the not seeing, Fi's tattoos and hangover – had got to me, and I felt hurt. It was the last audition I ever did. Interestingly, Aisha, an Indian-heritage South African teacher who I met in passing at a yoga studio several months later, told me she'd gone for a job at the Starbucks place too. Aisha believed she wasn't hired due to her ethnicity, because she had been the only person of colour trying out at the time – like I had. I couldn't know for sure if this was true, but how awful if it was. According to Aisha, Fi had said, 'You seem to know a lot about yoga and that's not quite what we're looking for,' when Aisha asked for feedback. I've never got to the bottom of what Fi was getting at when she said that.

Community and Sledgehammers

I'm on a video call, waiting for yoga teacher Norman Blair to arrive. I first met Norman in early 2016 shortly after stumbling across the nine-month Ashtanga and Yin teacher training run by him and fellow teacher Melanie Cooper that I later ended up doing. I was newly sober at the time so not feeling serious (or ready) to think about teaching. I was also still smoking (I had been advised to do one thing at a time and to focus on staying sober first) so didn't feel like the ideal candidate. But this course – the first I'd ever seen – on the practices I had devoted most of my time (and body and mind) to in recent years triggered an impulse to reach out. He encouraged me to enrol, but two weeks before it was due to start I got cold feet. I emailed to say I couldn't do it. But Norman encouraged me to go ahead. I'm grateful he did. Even if it meant that I had to find my excuses to leave the training studio at lunchtimes to chain-smoke as many roll-ups as I could in a nearby park.

Norman's an old-timer who has had a regular yoga practice since 1993 and started teaching in 2001. He is also the author of *Brightening our Inner Skies: Yin and Yoga*.[25] My favourite section in the book is the first half where he draws from his own experiences, challenges and upheavals in life to explore self-transformation and social responsibility (which you'll know by now are two things that interest me greatly). Norman and I are on the same page in lots of ways: we have to navigate our innate impulsiveness, we both have pasts with self-destructiveness and, perhaps most significantly, we both see politics in everything – including yoga. We also share the same rebellious tendency to push against the status quo.

'I wish more people had balls and could say what's going down. All of my adult life I've been involved in political things and I haven't been worried about speaking out,' Norman told me.

I remember going to my first political meeting when I was eighteen. I was getting arrested all the time. The first time was in 1983 when they brought cruise missiles into the UK from the US, but there were lots of occasions. And I was aware of my privileges. I remember getting stopped by police in the 1980s and I know that I got a much easier ride than, say, if I'd been Black.

We can claim yoga as being like a safety valve or a delusion that helps people feel a bit better but it's not as simple as that. One of the ways I view things is as an image of a disco ball with many angles. It's not yes or no; it's never binary. There are a whole load of situations and sides involved.

I wanted to know whether Norman's experience of yoga in the 1990s reflected mine since we both started practising during the same decade. 'It was much more low key when my regular practice started. There was a group of eight of us practising in someone's living room, which I think is a great way to learn. On Zoom I've taught very large events but there can be an issue there of putting someone on a pedestal. Then when you're on a pedestal it becomes a drug. You can easily start thinking: *I've got it all sorted out*, when the reality is that I'm as messed up as everyone else. So small groups are really healthy ways of going. You came along, did your practice; quite often we would have a cup of tea after. It was friendly. Then the commercialization of yoga arrived.'

Norman could easily be describing my own early classes at the YMCA and Ashtanga self-practise rooms over the years, where the groups were always small and we too would sometimes hang out, discuss our work and love lives or the perils of controversial spiritual leaders over coffee. I didn't see the scale of the commercialization happening under my nose. Where did it come from?

We need to look at Yoga Works in the US, which started in the early 1990s. Eventually they sold out to a group who sold out again and it got bigger and more corporate. In the early days of teaching Ashtanga in London, teachers all knew each other. Also, when I started teaching, there were fewer teachers so it was easier to find work. Now there is a lot of competition for classes and one of the consequences is that class pay rates have stayed the same or gone down. There has been a substantial reduction of pay in real terms from 2001 to 2020 and one of the only ways to earn more is by running teacher trainings. The problem with that is that just brings more people into an already saturated market. When I started teaching Yin in 2003, it was the only Yin class in London – and now there are hundreds. Which in some ways is wonderful. But I've wondered for a long time when the bubble is going to burst.

I asked if he thought it would.

I'm not sure. The 2020 COVID-19 pandemic was a puncture but the yoga industry just seems to keep getting bigger. Coming to teaching came out of a big personal upheaval for me when I needed to find work. I started teaching in gyms and leisure centres – much like you did. I saw it as an apprenticeship. It sorts the wheat from the chaff; you're only going there because you're interested in going to a gym rather than an expensive studio where they've got posh hand lotion. It was the same when I started going to Ashtanga Yoga London in 1999 at the Diorama Arts Centre where we were practising on office carpet. That's when Gwyneth Paltrow and Chris Martin were going there too. And I used to think: give them credit because they could easily have afforded to get someone to teach them on their shiny floorboards. But instead they were going to this place where there was no toilet paper sometimes.

Ah, I remember those humble days myself, before yoga became drenched in essential oils, wrapped in sweat-wicking active-wear and packaged with sound baths. Like Norman, I had my own apprenticeship in leisure centres. It felt like coalface work at times, but I learnt more in leisure centres than I have anywhere else because of the range of people, all the different bodies, the aches and pains, injuries, ages and difficult customers, and learning how to navigate the room and support everyone. It offered a big lesson in building relationships too, which is what teaching has always been about for me. And that's where yoga starts: with relationship to self, but then relationship to others, nature, and the world.

'The trouble is that a lot of people can get stuck in a relationship to self,' Norman told me. 'There can be a lot of self-absorption and narcissism. It's like the mat becomes a mirror to look at yourself. You might think: *wow, look how beautiful I am*, but one of the spin-offs is that narcissism is often a defence for low self-esteem. I'm not going to pretend I'm completely grounded – I'm not. But I've shifted a lot. I've done a lot of psychotherapy. I think every yoga teacher should see a psychotherapist – non-negotiable. Because when someone has that deep confidence in themselves, they don't have to stand up and talk about themselves. Whereas with a narcissistic person it's all very "look at me" because on some level they know there's a feeling of hollowness.'

This emptiness is why many of us end up in therapy. At least that was what seemed to be my big problem when I started analytical psychotherapy for the first time. I wasn't a narcissist, thankfully, but I discovered that the eating and drinking troubles, and possibly even the yoga classes I became obsessed with, filled an emptiness that I wasn't even aware of. It's perhaps what social media does too – where we look to strangers to applaud us, to fill an emptiness. The only reason I think Instagram didn't turn me into a narcissist (and, let's face it, it could easily have happened) is because the approval I got when I started growing a community online was mostly for things I had written or created about issues I deeply cared about. The mission and message felt more important than me. Like Norman, once I found my voice, I wanted to use it to uncover what I believed to be true.

One of the reasons I wanted to talk to Norman was to hear more about his part in the Yoga Teachers Union that was established in the UK in October 2020 to address the issue of pay and conditions for yoga teachers, which is something I had written about on Instagram before and had fallen on deaf ears. He says this about it:

Some of the things that drive me in life are about fairness and sustainability. It's about walking the talk. If I believe in fairness but then I notice people struggling to find work or receive a decent wage, I have to challenge it. My vision is that it's about having a space for teachers to discuss the issues we face and how we can improve things. So rather than me muttering away to you; it's about recognizing that other people are in a similar situation and working out what we can do about it.

On a personal level I do well from the training courses and workshops that I run. But what I see in the yoga world – which is a reflection of the rest of society – is one per cent of people doing really well. I feel a responsibility that if we see something that's wrong, we should try to make it better.

I told Norman that a friend of mine had to sign a non-disclosure agreement when she worked for a big studio brand in London, and his view was final: 'We should not be working anywhere that asks us to sign a non-disclosure agreement. I've had people tell me that they've had to teach twenty classes a week. I think this is bonkers. We talk about self-care but let's look in the mirror. The big studios need to wake up and think about how much they're caring for the people who are bringing in their custom. Yin teacher Bernie Clark in Canada talks about the Zen of running a business. It sees three different pillars: the owner, the customer and the worker. What's happened in the yoga industry is that there's a lot of attention paid to the customer, the owner has kept going and the teachers and receptionists have got stuffed.'

I asked Norman what he thought needed to happen for the yoga industry to improve its ethics, which it seems to me has to come from businesses taking care of its teachers.

'It might sound like I'm only on the side of the teachers but I'm also on the side of the studio. I have a strong memory of you, Nadia, once telling me that hashtags were going to change the world.' (Haha, it's true. I worked at a petitions platform at the time and that sounds like one of my media lines.)

'When you did, I probably didn't know what a hashtag was!' Norman continued. 'But I put a post on Facebook and I added #SupportYogaStudios. So I'm clear about supporting yoga studios, as long as they support teachers. Studios need to come back to this idea of the pillars. Obviously, we have to be financially realistic, but we have to prioritize sustainability.'

It feels like one of the biggest ironies of the wellness industry that businesses that are clearly thriving and making bucket loads of money choose not to invest some of that cash in their staff. It's certainly been the case for me and my experience of teaching in London. Why did this happen? I asked Norman.

I think part of the problem is that teachers teach because they love doing it but they are being exploited for it. So there's a sense of yoga of teachers being exploited for their love. We've come to yoga teaching out of our love for practice and then the studio, knowing that, thinks it doesn't need to pay us a fair wage.

This point about exploitation got me thinking about the endless teacher trainings churning out teachers who in some cases may be ill-equipped to teach or not have enough practice years under their belts before they start teaching. I generally have a knee-jerk reaction against regulation but I wonder whether there needs to be something in place, though I don't know what it would look like. Norman says:

Instinctively I'm against regulation too, but I do think yoga teachers need to be supervised. Psychotherapists are supervised. Why isn't there a similar setting for yoga teachers? I think we could all benefit from that kind of level of support. And sometimes you need to ask the question: why are you churning out so many teachers?

Where are the ethics? We saw this with the Pattabhi Jois scandal. Yoga teachers get a big investment in the system by being attached to a big name like his. That then made them reluctant to rock the boat, when actually the boat was sinking after the allegations of his abuse of women came out. The abuse was known, but people kept silent. Silence is violence because you're consenting. I think things need to be questioned more – in a loving and compassionate way – which in itself is quite challenging. The problem is that we live in an individualized society where it's sink or swim. Everyone feels like they've got to grab the life raft even though it's got an NDA attached to it. But actually it should be about us sitting down collectively and thinking about how we can improve the situation for everyone. The COVID-19 pandemic in 2020 gave us an opportunity. It was a sledgehammer to normality so I'm not going to say things will get better because they might get much worse. But there is a chance of shifting things. The question is: what are people going to do about it?

Norman's question is a powerful one that I think anyone involved in the business of yoga should think about. It's a question that led to me writing this book when I realized that teaching yoga wasn't what it was cracked up to be. At least, it hadn't been a smooth ride or lived up to its glossy appearance.

On the surface, yoga teaching had looked like a life of flying to exotic places, doing handstands on beaches and teaching classes in bougie gyms and studios. It looked like a glamorous and lucrative way to live but hadn't quite worked out that way for me because I didn't think yoga should be repurposed and commodified as it has been. Many people were benefiting from setting up yoga businesses or from teaching, but so many more like me were struggling to survive. At the same time I was thinking about the problem I saw, where yoga looked like it was being taken away from many people who might want to practise and not have access to it. The industry seemed to be taking yoga as I knew it away from me too, which isn't what I had expected when I started teaching yoga. I had hoped that teaching would have brought me closer to it. I suppose the big question I was wrestling with was, if I was going to survive as a yoga teacher and work in a way that I believed in, what was *I* going to do about it?

CHAPTER 9

When the Dream Dies

My conversation with Norman took me back to my early experiences of teaching and why I went into it in the first place. It also made me think back to the teacher training I did with him and Melanie in 2016. It had been my second attempt at teacher training, after the chaos in India several years earlier. On that first day with Norman and Melanie, the twelve of us on the course were asked to walk in a circle and take it in turns to step into the middle and introduce ourselves. When it got to my turn, I stepped up and instead of saying 'My name's Nadia and I'm a yoga teacher' as instructed, I said: 'Hi my name's Nadia and I hate this.' I just couldn't deal with being the only person speaking and everyone looking at me.

It was the same in our final assessment at a studio in West London. My mum had come to be one of the bodies in the classes we had to teach. 'What's happening to me?' I asked when I saw her come through the door and I held my shaking arms up to her face. 'It's adrenalin, eat these,' she told me, shoving a boxful of almonds into my trembling palms. When it was all over, I couldn't believe I had somehow managed to make it to the end of teaching a roomful of mostly strangers, let alone the nine-month course.

There had been so much to learn about anatomy, yoga philosophy, teaching techniques and theory that I struggled with the information overload at times. So why become a yoga teacher? Well, that hadn't been my plan. I'd gone on the training course because I wanted to deepen my learning of yoga, not for a spandex-wearing career change. Yoga has been a big part of my life for a long time. I liked the idea of sharing it, but the fear of public speaking was the biggest thing holding me back. I didn't want the limelight, plus I knew by then that I didn't look the part. Given the breadth and depth of yoga, I also questioned whether I was in fact yoga teacher material. Had I practised and worked on myself enough? Did I know who I was and understand yoga enough to share the practice? How would I live up to its puritanical image given my destructive past. I wasn't sure I could. Norman and Melanie both said they had 'every faith' in me. *Bet they say that to everyone*, I thought, but I decided to take their sentiments to heart and accepted that everyone has to start somewhere. Far more than any certificate, years of practising yoga seemed to be as good a starting point as any.

Once I started teaching a couple of years later, I was still scared of standing at the front of the room but there was something else going on too. As I saw other teachers at yoga job interviews and auditions, I noticed how self-assured they were. Where did they get that confidence from, I'd wonder? I felt imposter syndrome creeping in. This bundle of insecurity, apprehension and uncertainty quickly turned to outright anxiety when I started teaching full-time. The anxiety kept getting bigger when I began using social media to advertise my classes. I didn't relate to the images I saw of ambitious yoga teachers and practitioners performing intricate and complex poses. I found the images I saw intimidating even after more than two decades of practising yoga. Despite flicking through endless social media posts overlaid with pretty fonts quoting Persian poet Rumi or captions reassuring me that I was 'enough' – I didn't think I was. I wanted to feel I belonged more than anything, because yoga meant so much to me. But these posts didn't reflect me. If these yogis with their agile bodies, huge social media followings and overwhelmingly positive got-everything-sussed outlooks were what it meant to be a yoga teacher, well I had strong doubts on whether I would ever measure up.

And I'd really tried.

When I first started teaching, I bought a pile of new multi-coloured leggings and tops in an online shopping spree. The plan was to build a teaching wardrobe so I would look the part and therefore be taken seriously. 'What do you think?' I asked James after I had pulled on a baggy white tank top with glow-stick green neckline. 'Nice?' I probed. It looked like something from a rave in the 1990s, but I liked it. 'It's not very teacher-y is it?' was his not-quite-what-I-was-looking-for response.

'But I don't want to look like a teacher, I still want to look like me,' I wailed, yanking it off and storming out of the bedroom. The thing is – I did. I desperately wanted to look like a yoga teacher. I wished I was flexible enough to do the splits, get my leg behind my head, and longed to be able to do all the advanced hand-balancing poses that they could. I wanted a flatter stomach, stronger hand-standing arms, and to float through sequences as they did. I'd been doing so many of these poses for years – longer than a lot of new yoga teachers I met – and felt short-changed that I couldn't go deeper in back bends or hold a handstand without a wall. That would make me look more teacher-y, wouldn't it? And when you don't feel the part at least you can look at the part, I would tell myself.

So I kept trying.

I had noticed on the teaching circuit that, when I walked in to cover another teacher's class in their absence, I was often faced with expectant yoga practitioners who wanted elaborately choreographed sequences set to upbeat soundtracks. It was nerve-wracking and it wasn't how I practised, but I obliged, spending hours designing classes and crafting playlists (when I believed people should really be listening to their breath instead). I wouldn't sleep the night before teaching a new group. I'd lie there, rehearsing sequences in my mind. I'd force James to walk through the moves with me at home, and scribble notes on the back of my hand to revise on the way to teaching. If my brain went blank I'd glance down at my hand when everyone was in Downward Facing Dog Pose (and they can't see you) to confirm what we might do next.

It felt wrong. I was conflicted between the studio owners' and students' expectations and the desire to share a practice that I loved in a way that felt true to me. This is what I had assumed I would be doing. But I couldn't escape the heavy pressure to entertain and perform. It felt to me as though you had to have a certain kind of personality as a yoga teacher, a wellness script to live by, and – given my past with eating disorders and alcoholism, the numerous walk-outs on yoga and giving up on it – I wasn't sure I measured up after all. What I was seeing for the first time looked to me like a one-size-fits-all influencer model of how yoga teachers should behave and promote themselves. Of course, there are lots of teachers not behaving in this way, but I'm talking about the dominant culture as it appeared to me in the circles that I found myself in. I wasn't up for it. It was killing the spirit of yoga. It took a year of teaching full-time before I found the confidence to teach in a way that I felt aligned more with my own experience of yoga. Even then the pressure to jazz up classes and make them more funky would creep back in.

Yoga is a holistic system that's often talked about as a method for unifying mind and body. My understanding of this in simple terms is that we practise so that we might get to a place where there is no body, nor mind. In a sense this might mean that we meditate until we find nothing there. The aim with practice is to become aligned with the essence of who we are. I'm endlessly fascinated by this and still have no idea what it is that makes me who I am. But imagine feeling that kind of connection with your true self – whatever that is. How might life be? It's this search for that elusive thing that I think has made me stick with yoga for so long. This idea that we practise to get to a place where the self transcends the material self of mind and body as an absolute entity. So the posture-heavy yoga we see everywhere has its place – and I love the poses – but it shouldn't stop there. Taking yoga simply as an exercise class – or what I call *yoga-cise* – isn't going to allow that to happen.

I had a turning point after teaching for a couple of years, when I started to wonder whether what I had been doing was a mistake. I loved sharing the practice, so the individual classes I taught weren't the problem. It was the wider industry that was revealing itself to me that was starting to make me feel uncomfortable. It felt like it might be time to quit teaching altogether. I reduced the number of classes

I was teaching and started working full-time as head of front of house at a yoga studio. Bad move. I left after four months.

James, who was used to me making impulsive decisions, suggested I stick it out a while longer to make sure I was doing the right thing, but life had become awful and I couldn't. On my last day I sat on a bench at a train station and reflected. At moments of leaving or arriving, the past comes into relief vividly, and I started thinking about mine. I was in my late thirties, jobless and without a plan – again. As I looked down the empty station platform, I knew that I would have to take responsibility for what had happened, somehow muddle through and work out where I should head next. Life is about the journey, so the saying goes, but if you don't have a rough idea of a destination how are you supposed to get there?

I had been ambivalent about discovering what lay beneath the earnest surface of yoga when I applied for the yoga studio job, which had opened its doors only months earlier. But I also had high hopes. When you've practised yoga as long as I have, it seems natural to want to work in it full-time. I also thought that I could make a difference from the inside. I might be able to influence hiring processes, get a diverse workforce in place, and in turn attract a broader demographic of the community like I had seen in the leisure centres. I tried, but with the little power I had, the reality didn't match the dream.

Do what you love, and you'll never work a day in your life.

I used to see this painted on walls in a WeWork flexible office when I worked in a communications job. It felt like what I had tried to do, but it hadn't worked out. Because what I loved (yoga) looked like it was being destroyed. *Find something to love about what you do* might have been a more realistic approach. A steady income is what had seduced me when I took the studio job. I had been struggling to earn enough as a yoga teacher, was burnt out from spending so much of my time on public transport and hustling for teaching gigs to make ends meet. But the twist in this tale is that working at a wellness company had left me feeling exceptionally unwell.

A month into working there James, whose flat I'd moved into by then, had been saying things like: 'Babe, you're angry all the time,' and 'I think you might need help.' He meant it was time to find a therapist. This was after I'd kicked off another 'you don't understand' argument before leaving the flat, saying 'I'm going for a walk.' I wasn't used to being angry all the time, and I didn't know why I was. I seemed to be permanently anxious. The anxiety was mixed with a quiet rage at the yoga that I was complicit in selling.

The irony that the yoga industry is dominated by white teachers perpetuating a culture around the Western interpretation of yoga wasn't lost on me. It made me question whether I was overreacting and wrong to feel conflicted. *I should live and let live*, I would try to reason with myself. *Just ignore it and do it your way*, I would say. But really I was gaslighting myself. *It's all in your head, you're just not made for this, call yourself a yoga teacher?* was what my brain was telling me in the way it often does when you're not sure how you have ended up where you are.

But I couldn't help but see that what was happening around me was a perverse form of twenty-first-century colonialism. This paradox soon became exhausting to exist within. Here I was, feeling forced to distort and rebrand a tradition that was not what I understood it to be. I didn't feel that yoga belonged to me because of my South Asian heritage any more than it did to anyone else, but it did make me wonder what my place should be within all of this. I wondered if the students I taught noticed what I saw as an unusual reverse of power in classes, with me usually being the only person of colour in the room, not least the person calling the shots and telling everyone what to do. I tried not to let this get to me, but it did. I wanted to see more people of colour in my classes so that I wouldn't feel outnumbered myself. Seeing yourself reflected in others, even if they don't share the same cultural background, means you relax somewhere on an inexplicable level. That joint 'otherness' is what connects you. It's a feeling of recognition, of shared experience.

I consoled myself that other people of colour might feel inspired to take up yoga and feel welcome in classes, by seeing me around. But it didn't seem to make much difference and I felt lonely. The students in my classes remained predominantly white. Whenever a person of colour did turn up, we clocked each other, and I always enjoyed teaching the class more.

The longer I spent in the job at the studio, the more on edge I felt. It didn't help that I met a lot of yoga teachers who came out with things that put me in a bad mood. One told me that she was convinced she had Indian genes because she liked squatting. *Wait, what?!* Had I heard that right? She wafted away before I could respond. Not that I would have known what to say. I sat on the front desk for the rest of the day, trying to work out why I was annoyed. Was it fair of me to be? Or was what she said racist? I couldn't tell, but comments like that which left me speechless came to be common during my time in that job. They made me feel like no one could see who I was. I think it is called 'spiritual bypassing' these days. I felt invisible although I knew I stood out because I was one of the only people of colour in the building most of the time.

It was as though I was teetering on the edge of a nervous breakdown but not quite having it. I had noticed a pattern in my mood swings several months after I stopped drinking. They were frequent and more extreme than before. I thought that with eighteen months of sobriety under my belt – around about the time I started working at the studio – life would be different, but no. I felt thin-skinned and had underestimated how fragile the recovery process can make one feel. Healing hurts. I had only gone five months without a drink when I met James. I felt on top of things and ready for a relationship because I had achieved the unthinkable and stopped drinking. But as our years together went by, I was still restless: hurtling from one job to the next, from one internal conflict to the next life crisis. I was a minefield and he happened to be the first person to walk into it.

Despite the angst it caused me, the yoga studio job did serve a purpose in my life. I didn't like the funky decor, classes on offer or indeed the self-important clientele it seemed to attract, but I'm grateful for the experience because it confirmed that a lot of the inner churning I'd been feeling after I started to teach yoga had been legitimate.

The studio itself was on a busy main road filled with second-hand electronic shops, supermarket chains, everything-for-a-quid discount stores, new vegan cafes and older greasy spoons that now proudly stocked oat milk. Through the glass front of the building, passers-by could see the front desk where I spent most of my time. The studio was new, so the locals were still getting used to it being there and would frequently stop and stare, noses almost pressed up to the glass. I wondered what everyone made of it. I also questioned how many of the people in the area the studio would serve and which of them would be able to afford it.

On opening night, you had to hand it to the yogi-preneur owners for their optimism. Earlier, I'd got to the space at midday and it was covered in sawdust with builders, electricians and a bloke trying to sort the internet line out. The front desk was littered with toolbox debris, bottles of Lucozade, biscuits, Rizlas and fat pouches of tobacco. I was surprised by the number of people who came on the first night. We had no electricity, so no lights, heating or Wi-Fi. I stood behind the front desk, signing people in via a phone app. The improvised, seemingly ordered chaos of that first night illustrates a microcosm of the yoga world at large. It might look polished but there are a lot of creaky floorboards beneath those promises of tranquillity. Everything that had made me apprehensive about working at a yoga studio (because it would mean I'd see it for what it truly was) came true. Things can look slick and serene on the surface, especially in the new world of yoga we find ourselves in today. But the truth is, everyone's winging it.

Halfway through the evening, the owner went to the pub with some of the building crew. He came back shortly before closing and collapsed exhausted on a beanbag. I felt the same. I hung around for an hour after the last class finished at 9 p.m., trying to tidy up as much as anyone can in the dark. Afterwards, I stepped into the bitter January night to go home. It felt like it was going to be a long first month. It was.

Four months later I was done with it. I reached out to one of my yoga mentors to check I wasn't going mad. I told them everything that was bothering me. About the studio where I was still working, and fresh sexual abuse allegations coming out against too many so-called gurus that had forced yoga to face its own #MeToo crisis. I explained some of the problematic issues – specifically what I was seeing with cultural appropriation, glib 'Namaslay all day' slogans on expensive T-shirts, the narcissism of some teachers. And how, at auditions, I was almost always the only person of colour trying out in a crowd of white faces. The sad fact was that none of this was surprising anymore. Yoga is meant to help me feel balanced and clear-headed, but all it was doing was making me feel very wobbly. I was feeling very sorry for myself.

'It feels like there's less integrity in yoga than there should be,' I said. I didn't mean in the practice itself but the industry surrounding it. 'What shall I do?' My wise mentor, who admitted these were not times in which they themselves would want to be a new teacher, advised that it might be time to 'step away from the froth'. The froth was all of the above, along with the social media-fication of yoga, teachers becoming celebrities and presenting us at worst with a tyrannous, quasi-ideological lifestyle that we should all want to be living. A week after that meeting with my mentor, I went home in tears for no apparent reason after a long shift at the studio again. I resigned the next day.

My boss had been shocked when I said I wanted to go, which was understandable, since I had clearly been doing a good job hiding my real feelings. He phoned me immediately after receiving my resignation email. Did I want more money? What had happened? He wanted to know. 'It's just not the right fit. No hard feelings,' I lied, hiding in one of the showers in the women's changing room and hoping a customer wouldn't walk in and see me. I was disappointed. If I couldn't hack it as a yoga teacher or as a staff member in a popular yoga studio I had no idea what I was going to do.

I was waking up to a modern version of yoga that I was now working within and I hated it. I was stressed and depressed – all the time. Cracks had also been showing up beyond that yoga studio within the wider wellness industry, which looked pretty ill to me, too. That's why I left.

At the station on my last day at that job, I stepped onto a train, thinking I should feel excited. I was free to go anywhere. *I should go and do something crazy to mark this moment,* I thought. But all I really wanted to do was to go home. As I stared at my phone, a message came through from a friend. 'Are you a free woman again?' it said. I was, but I felt bruised, let down and possibly heartbroken. I knew that I would need to take it easy for a while to recover. *I should probably forget about life plans and designs and just let things ebb and process through for a while*, I thought. But that's the big trouble, I've never found that easy: if I close one door, I'm anxious to fling another open immediately.

I felt that I had done the right thing, that nothing good would have come from staying in that job. The owners were better off with someone who believed in their business, which I realized I didn't. It also occurred to me that the experience of that job was an aperture into something much bigger: the crystallization of what yoga had become and was fast turning into, something shinier yet uglier than yoga as I'd known it for the past twenty-five years, a sometimes-soulless business selling the promise of healing for the soul. It had become something I didn't recognize: a kind of Yoga Industrial Complex – a giant hungry machine pumping out T-shirts bearing Om symbols and hands in a prayer position. Why did yoga have to be this way? My dreams had been shattered, but the bigger problem was down to what working as a teacher and within the yoga studio had symbolized: the unthinking clichés they adopted, and the entire Nike-ified lifestyle they seemed part of.

Seeing the yoga business from the inside made me question everything. *What was I doing here? Why hadn't I seen this before?* I realized I didn't believe in 'the yoga business' – or really, what happens when something that feels like it shouldn't be a business is turned into one. Particularly when it's ripped from its roots, cleansed, perfumed and commodified, repackaged in pretty pastels with decontextualized Sanskrit. Yoga was starting to feel like a lie. I was lost in a wellness maze and was going to have to find a way out.

Through thick and thin, illness and wellness in the truest sense of the word, yoga had been a constant in my life for a long time – a steady friend that has always been there when I've been ready to return to it. But working within it had made me feel like yoga might have become my worst enemy or at least something I was in a painful relationship with. I was starting to wonder if I hated yoga.

CHAPTER 10

The Ashtangover

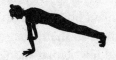

I knew that the yoga studio job couldn't be blamed for everything that went wrong for me on my yoga teaching journey, but it shone a spotlight on fragilities I was already feeling. It also fully exposed problems I was seeing in the yoga world. As stressed out as it left me, it simply confirmed that much of the inner churning I'd been feeling after I started teaching yoga had been valid. Teaching had been throwing up insecurities (*am I good enough to do it?*), inner conflicts (*I don't fit in . . .*) and anger (*what the hell has happened to yoga?*), which the management job only amplified. It also revealed more comprehensively to me that yoga had lost its way.

I couldn't change the industry and it was obvious to me that I didn't fit in, but there was something stopping me from turning my back on it too. I decided to take my mentor's advice to step away from the froth and think about what I could do to keep teaching but in a way I was happy about. I started doing what my mum had suggested when I had got myself in a state after all the auditions I had been on: I focused on my own practice. It had worked at tricky times before so I figured that it would work now. What had happened wasn't important; all that mattered was what was right in front of me, which was another crossroads with no clear path in sight.

I continued practising Ashtanga at home and started exploring Dharma Yoga with the 'practise each pose as a prayer' teacher (on page 103) at a studio. Within a few weeks, calm was restored. As usual, focusing on my own practice created the space I needed to listen to my heart and I knew what to do. I realized that when I boiled everything down, I liked the main aspect of teaching: to share a practice I loved. I had to find a way to keep doing it that didn't cause me so much anxiety. I started looking for new places to teach again and by the summer of 2019 I was teaching regularly at several studios where I developed strong relationships with the owners. I felt safe and happy working in this way, which made me more discerning about the jobs I took. I decided that I only wanted to work with people I got on with and liked. I didn't want to go back out to auditions, so I had to find another way to get work.

Slowly I started to teach private clients in their homes, and teaching in some workplaces followed. I was teaching less because I stopped covering as many classes as I had before and I felt happier. My fear of public speaking also finally left by working in this new way – yoga teaching cured me of that in the end. I was still struggling to earn enough to get by but I had to stick to my guns and not get roped into teaching classes I didn't want to. I got an evening job in a Pakistani restaurant kitchen to top up my income. I prepared orders and became an expert at making fifty rotis over a shift, which was laughable to me at first because I had never made a roti that was edible or round in my life until then. It was hot and hard work. An eight-hour shift paid the same as what I might have got for teaching a private client and it was tiring. But life got better and I felt I had landed on my feet. Then, just as I was starting to feel settled, the COVID-19 pandemic hit the UK, which would change the course of my relationship with yoga again, and I started talking publicly about it.

Yoga in the Time of Corona

I've often joked to friends that getting sober and stopping smoking were the best and worst things I've ever done. Best because . . . well, that's obvious: improved health. Worst because it means regular confrontation with the way I feel. It's the same with yoga. Once I started seeing the problems, I couldn't un-see or stop thinking about them. I dealt with this by writing posts on social media. I wrote lengthy pieces about the big problems that I saw when yoga has been distorted into something that it wasn't. 'The old yoga was intended to be about self-discovery and meditation, while the new practice we have today appears to have become a self-serving, fitness-focused, trendy, expensive, and in many ways elitist activity,' I told my 400 or so followers. No one was interested. But everything changed when the UK first went into lockdown in March 2020.

Those early weeks of the pandemic were unsettling times for everyone across the world as we adjusted to socially distant lives. All my teaching work dried up immediately, so I was jobless again, and after a few days of dragging myself onto my mat each morning and then having no plans, I got tired of improvising my life every day. I needed structure. I missed the regular yoga students I used to teach and practising in a room with others.

It felt like, in its own disastrous way, COVID-19 had happened because the world was spinning too fast, our existing actions hurting ourselves, others and the planet. It couldn't go on like that. Nature in its own catastrophic way was forcing us to change urgently. It felt like global devastation, paving the way for a rebirth. But it was too much for me. I was restless, irritable and my relationship with James was on edge. Being cooped up meant that I thought about alcohol a lot and on other days felt disorientated around food. I wasn't moving as much as I was used to due to being housebound, which confused me and I didn't know if I was eating too much. If I had toast in the morning, could we order a pizza in the evening? It might sound ridiculous but that's what disordered eating in my experience is – nonsensical. I couldn't make sense of anything, and food is the default setting that I switch back to when highly anxious or stressed, even more so since I stopped drinking.

Outside our home, the world's grind to a halt seemed to be inspiring many people to take a contemplative look at their lives and reinvent their approaches. In those early weeks I think I saw more adverts for yoga mats, pants and bras than I did for online Zoom yoga classes. It was fascinating to watch how the impact of coronavirus left us all feeling so emotionally fragile and how that in turn led to a boom in online and live-streamed yoga. Other workouts went online too but there seemed to be a particular interest in yoga. I wondered what my place should be in all of this.

I resisted teaching online for as long as possible because I still didn't want to be part of the 'yoga scene'. It didn't take long before I changed my mind and started running my own classes via Zoom after several old students asked if I would. I needed something to do and I realized that if it would help others for me to step up (as well as earn some money), then I should find a way to do it. I offered drop-in classes every morning and moved my private clients online. I started teaching my mum as a way to check in with her every week, and a friend who was quarantined in Thailand as well as her mother in France. It took a while to get used to but luckily my classes were small so I could build relationships with the new faces who came. I couldn't imagine what it would have been like to teach a huge class full of strangers, which was what many other teachers were doing. I would see them post pictures to social media of their Zoom galleries filled with tiny squares.

Teaching online occupied me for a while, helped build walls around my day and I grew to enjoy it. At the same time, it got me thinking about how many people would stick with a practice once lockdown restrictions were lifted. Or indeed look into the deeper meaning behind yoga. *That'll show us how deep this new uptake is going to go*, I thought. I hoped people would stick to it, but I was pent up with cabin fever and sceptical. This is when, sitting on the sofa after teaching one morning as I scrolled mindlessly through Instagram, I had an idea. Earlier in the year I had written a piece for *HuffPost* called 'Why I'm Not Talking to White People about Yoga'[26] (the headline was inspired by Reni Eddo-Lodge's excellent book about race[27]). It was my first public comment on the state of modern yoga and summarized key things that had started getting me down since I began teaching yoga. It got quite the response. Some people loved it and told me they were grateful to me for speaking out, but trolls who couldn't get past the headline said it was offensive and clickbaity. I was accused of being racist (nope) and told to go back to South Asia (this is what racism sounds like).

With all the extra time I had on my hands in lockdown, I started sharing my views on the yoga industry on social media again and this time took a more aggressive approach.

I experimented by making mini-vlogs talking about cultural appropriation, what I saw as a problem with crash-course yoga teacher training and the entire Instagramification of yoga and wellness. Everything that had been building up inside me in previous years came pouring out. I lost followers and panicked as I was already unemployed and thought no one would want to hire me in future if I got a reputation for being shouty. But anxiety propelled me on, and I couldn't stop. I posted a video about the misuse of the yoga industry's favourite word, Namaste, and that's when things blew up. My main argument was that it was a Hindu greeting and had nothing to do with yoga. Dozens of people shared it and thousands of people watched it, which at the time was the biggest impact anything I had posted had ever had.

I had struck a chord. So I kept going. My private messages were on fire. South Asians got in touch to tell me that they felt seen and thanked me for putting into words how they had been feeling and why they had been put off attending yoga classes. Other teachers across the world said that they felt empowered to tell their own stories and raise conversations on similar issues in their communities. I couldn't believe it. What had I stumbled upon here? I didn't quite know but, after navigating these thoughts on my own for so long and all the lonely years of teaching and struggling with my feelings, I felt like I had finally found my voice. I could now talk freely about everything I wanted to, because there were people who wanted to listen.

What happened for me through Instagram was significant because it revealed that what I was speaking about mattered to me personally but also more importantly resonated with others. I wasn't alone. At the same time, finding my voice led to the *yoga dissident* moniker I had chosen – something that started as an off-hand thing, a joke – to take on a genuine meaning. I had become a dissident to yoga at the same time as I loved the practice. I was declaring myself publicly as a nonconformist to the yoga industry due to my punk-esque refusal to be part of the mainstream and my desire to expose truths. After all, 2020 was a year when the entire world had to face big truths, and someone had to say all this stuff even if going against the mainstream is a lonely path at times. The more I posted, the larger my online community grew and the yoga manifesto started revealing itself to me.

Within a couple of weeks, I was invited to participate in Instagram Live (IG Live) talks and podcasts, and I said yes to everything because I was so happy that people were interested. Then George Floyd was murdered by police in the US. I was distraught. I couldn't focus on anything but his murder, the state of racism in America, in the UK and, it must be said, online. I felt powerless and didn't know what to do so I hosted an online class to raise money for Black Lives Matter in the UK and then I took a break from teaching. I didn't have the heart for it. James and I spent several days wandering around the flat, unable to talk about anything else. 'When is this going to stop?' I asked him. 'I'm angry and I'm sad and I don't know what to do,' I told him, sobbing into my hands. 'I don't want to be angry all the time again,' I said. 'We should be angry,' was all he could say. I felt relieved that I was in a relationship with someone who felt the same way. We sat at each end of the sofa holding hands, holding our anger, crying together.

In the weeks following Floyd's murder, I flashed back to my days as a crime reporter, when almost all the murders I wrote about were of Black boys. I thought about the grieving mothers who invited me into their homes and gave me photographs of their children, trusting me to do a good job in a tribute piece. I recalled the trainers I would see outside bedrooms belonging to sons who weren't coming home, and the mother who told me she would still wait to hear her son's key in the door. I wasn't a journalist anymore, but I felt compelled to do what I've done longer than I've done anything in my life: tell stories about the issues that matter. I thought about my position and what it meant for me to be an anti-racist ally, and I took the opportunity to interrogate the wellness space further than I had done before. I started applying the yoga principles of non-violence, truthfulness and self-study to what I saw going on in the world around me. I wrote a blog on my website where I coined the term Engaged Yoga. It was inspired by Thích Nhất Hạnh's idea of Engaged Buddhism, which he created during the Vietnam War. Engaged Buddhism is about practising in order to be aware of what's going on, he explains. If Buddhism isn't engaged, then it's not real Buddhism. I felt the same about yoga. This is an extract from what I wrote[28]:

> *Yoga is a practice for self-inquiry that allows us to learn about ourselves, connect with what we believe in, choose what values we're aligned with and decide who we're going to stand up for. This is what I call Engaged Yoga, and it's the only yoga I believe in.*
>
> *We must practise so that we're resilient and then we must go out and do the important work of the world. Engaged Yoga for me involves standing against inequalities amongst all people – and principally racism. I don't mean simply identifying passively as non-racist, I mean being vocally and actively anti-racist. The perverse hatred and oppression and murder of Black people which unthinkably still goes on has to stop. This isn't just a Black problem. It isn't just an American*

problem. It's all of our problem. And if we're not Black, we have privilege and have got to use it.

The Ahimsa (non-violence) tenet of yoga philosophy dictates not being violent to yourself or anyone else. This appears to get repackaged as #selfcare by the wellness industry. But what's the point of self-care if we're not using the strength and self-knowledge we cultivate to also care for others? We must practise for the world. People talk about how yoga must evolve with the changing times. This tends to mean mixing up postures, adding playlists and sprinkling on a heavy dose of good vibes only. For me real evolved yoga is a yoga that's involved in looking closely at ourselves and being engaged in the world around us, doing what we can to end suffering. For me a big part of this is fighting racism and campaigning against the murder of Black people. Because Black lives matter.

Ignorant people like to spout: 'All Lives Matter'. But this is wrong. White lives have always mattered. Black lives matter, because we live in a world where white supremacy (a racist ideology) means that they don't. It's not Ahimsa – and your yoga means nothing if you ignore this. And ignorance is a choice.

I meant for my blog to be a call to action, urging anyone involved in yoga to think about what their practice meant in terms of their place in the world. The idea resonated with many and it gave me hope that change might be coming. My piece was shared and reposted hundreds of times and I felt driven on by the support. It felt like an even more important piece than the one I had written in *HuffPost*, and I wasn't going to back down now. Neither were other people who were having their own awakenings about yoga and how a shift in the way things were done was needed.

I started seeing a huge wave of online discussions, IG Lives, posts and articles about cultural appropriation in yoga and how diversity suddenly mattered, and looked on as more people joined the conversation. Then newsletters started hitting my inbox from wellness businesses admitting that 'more needs to be done' to improve diversity within their workplaces. But because I had been trying to raise these conversations before Floyd's murder this new interest made me ask the questions: What are you going to do? How long is it going to take? And why didn't you do it before?

It seemed odd to me that some people were suddenly interested in racism as though it was a new problem – such as a global pandemic – that had come along. Further I was surprised that many yoga teachers of colour on social media appeared to be happy about the new interest in diversity and representation as if we finally had permission to talk about it. This is what pained me the most, because when I had raised these issues before, no one had been listening. Also, it felt that diversity was what everyone latched onto and I didn't buy it. Changing the ethnic wallpaper of yoga websites to include the faces of people of colour wasn't going to shake up the industry in the way it needed. It felt like a smokescreen when the marketing suddenly had more diverse representation yet the yoga being sold was still exclusive, expensive and culturally appropriated. Representation matters, of course, but it won't fix the wellness industry's colossal problems alone. The support for my work grew as I took a different turn in what I shared. While before I had been focused on critiquing and calling out yoga's problems, I now felt that I had found my mission: changing the narrative of yoga as a practice for wellness and #selfcare to calling on practitioners to look closely at why they practise and asking teachers to interrogate why they teach.

My experience on social media wasn't all a stroll through the park, sadly. After the initial surge of support, I got trolled too – in pernicious ways that had a disastrous effect on my mental health. The trouble was that I was being trolled and I didn't know it was trolling until it was too late. It came to a head when what looked like Hindu nationalists came after me around International Yoga Day when I wrote a strong post attacking Indian Prime Minister Modi's politics. I felt that I had pushed things too far and that everyone hated me, because the attacks were a relentless barrage of misogyny, homophobia and Islamophobia for several days. I couldn't cope. I was new to this kind of online exposure and ill-equipped to deal with it. Some of my new followers were kind enough to stick up for me but nothing could stop my anxiety, which kept growing, and the trolls meant that I was crying every day. I became manic, neurotic, and I was impossible to live with, obsessively checking updates on my screen, unable to ignore anything coming in. The trolling got so bad that I accidentally deleted my Instagram account. All the posts and videos I had spent hours preparing and writing disappeared. It was a big shock and felt as though I didn't exist anymore. But in a way that was what I had wanted – to delete myself, or the version of myself that I was showing the world. I had wanted all the noise to go away but I hadn't meant to do that.

My relationship broke down under these pressures. James couldn't deal with my unpredictable moods anymore and asked me to move out. I didn't see that coming. The union that I had dreamily thought would last for ever had snapped in two. It felt like he had given up on us. I couldn't handle that and my world fell apart. I lived at a friend's place out of a suitcase for a couple of months in what felt like purgatory while I found somewhere else to live, largely in denial about what my life had come to. I moved into a studio flat and tried to work out what had gone wrong. I was heartbroken and my life felt like it had burned down around me. I had never lived alone before; I felt lonely and injured. I would drag myself onto my yoga mat each morning, and half-heartedly move through the postures. My breath was all over the place, my chest tight like there was a padlock over my heart.

I thought often about something Thích Nhất Hạnh has said: that when animals in the forest are injured they rest. They know that to stop is to allow healing to take place, which human beings often fail to do.[29] I couldn't rest. I was agitated and confronted by those big questions again: *Why am I still doing this? Do I still believe in this practice? Is it going to help this time?* I wasn't sure.

As I navigated my new loveless existence, I learnt a big lesson about the need for boundaries in one's life. My experience of social media had made me insecure, destroyed my sense of self and killed the only relationship I'd ever wanted to last. Lockdowns across the world had been attempts by governments to stall the chaos of the outside world but I'd created another tornado inside myself. The disorder that first roused its head in my rebellious school days clearly hadn't left me. I fell into a bulimia relapse. I didn't know why. I hadn't been sick for many years.

'What the hell is wrong with me?' I complained to my therapist over a Zoom call. 'Why has this come back?' I didn't expect him to understand when I couldn't make sense of it myself.

'What has helped before?' he wanted to know. I couldn't remember but somehow my food problems had sorted themselves out when I got sober because I had enough to deal with going through that. Then I met James and it was as if our relationship cured me. I'd cook massive bowls of colourful food, trying out recipes, mixing textures and flavours and adding chilli to everything. I loved cooking for us both and we enjoyed eating together. That's what I lost when we broke up. I realized that eating alone was something I had hated all my life, and this felt like part of the reason I couldn't do it now. Until James left me, I had never understood that when people say they can't stomach something, what they mean is the thing in question is too overwhelming for them to confront. Through talking to my therapist, I realized that I couldn't stomach the pain of my break-up and in turn couldn't handle digesting food once again. I learnt that I was struggling to sit with a full stomach because I was already full of emotions that I couldn't identify, find the words for or accept.

It was as obvious as that, but knowing why I was relapsing wasn't enough to help me stop. It was my first relapse since I stopped drinking. I fantasized about the day I would be free but the statistics are not good. According to UK eating-disorder charity Beat, research suggests that 46 per cent of anorexia patients fully recover and 20 per cent remain chronically ill. Similar research into bulimia suggests that 45 per cent make a full recovery and 23 per cent suffer chronically.[30] A year later I still missed James and my symptoms were worse. I couldn't go on like this. I told my therapist what was going on. I was surprised that he wasn't in a hurry to make me keep a food diary like Cognitive Behavioural Therapists have done in my past.

'I've got a mental illness, haven't I?' I wailed. 'I'm mentally ill. There's a monster living inside me. It's like computer malware stuck in my body and I don't know how it got there. I'm going to be one of those people who never gets well.' I really meant it. I felt lost. I had spent a long time plagued by food but having so many years of recovery stacked up behind me made the pain of relapse unbearable.

My therapist was unfazed. 'This is a regression,' he told me. 'There's no need to panic. Everything that's happened has been destabilizing. You're struggling to process how you feel. What happened with James has been a huge trauma. You both had a lot there. It's a loss, an abandonment, and I know you're not going to like this but it's a re-enactment of that early rejection from your dad.'

Not my dad again, I thought. *Why does everyone (ex-boyfriends, this therapist, my mum) keep bringing it up?* But I knew deep down that there was no point in arguing with him when I was desperate to feel better.

'But why have I been attacking my body all my life? My poor body I've put through so much.' I paused and felt hollow with sadness. I couldn't deal with it so kept talking. 'I should know how to take care of myself by now. I hate my body and I hate that I hate it. I'm obviously a bad feminist.'

And this is where he said something I wish I had known years ago. 'You're okay, Nadia. You're not falling apart and you're not bad,' he told me. 'There's no static goodness or badness in anyone. Eating disorders are one of the most complex issues we deal with as therapists. They aren't anti-feminist. You're demolishing your body, denying it of pleasure, or eating too much without any pleasure. This is too often reduced to the idea of being thin. It's not as simple as that. It's not about size but about an inability to metabolize emotions. It's to do with suppressing a female body, or forcing it to stay in a childlike state. So we must ask why. This is the work we have to do together.'

Everything he said made sense, but it also sounded like a long process. I just wanted to stop being sick right now. I was frustrated that my therapist didn't have a quick-fix solution and thought he was wrong about me not falling apart: I felt like I already had. Unlike my teenage years of disordered eating, when I was binging and vomiting several times a day, I was managing to eat, albeit in a very structured and rigid way. On the outside I probably looked normal, but on the inside I'd confused my digestive system so much that I was uncomfortable every time anything solid hit my stomach and emotionally I didn't know how to keep it in. I felt like I was in disguise. I scrolled through social media, staring at body positive activists and others who had turned their backs on eating disorders and were thriving. I wanted to be like them. I've never been body positive and yet I've had a body that apparently blends into mainstream culture. Somewhere along the way – maybe it was yoga, or finding myself in happier times in my life – I seemed to get better. Was part of me now refusing to get well even though it was the thing I was desperate to achieve? I had obviously never recovered before and had simply been in remission for the years I had been well. The illness had tricked me.

How had I ended up here? I would ask myself every day. *Who even was I? When would I know?* Which got me wondering if I ever *would* know. Should I know? Do we ever really know who we are? I tried to make sense of what was behind my latest destruction. It didn't feel like an obsession with body shape or flesh this time; there was a bigger fear that I couldn't put my finger on. The evening meals were the hardest. But a year of relapse was enough. I had hit rock bottom months before. I was on my knees then but, as I had done previously, I kept getting back up again, falling down and getting up to keep going. I bought a juicer, thinking I should cleanse myself inside out, which goes against all the advice from nutritional experts who generally agree detoxes are best avoided by anyone who has a history of disordered eating even if they are now well. I didn't listen. I thought a few days of giving my stomach a rest would sort everything out. Two days of nothing but juices was enough before I was so hungry that I had to eat a banana. As soon as I ate any more I had to be sick. So my solution was to keep juicing and then I got hooked on it. *Why do I always get addicted to everything?* I later tried one liquid day a week and was eating too much and throwing up for the rest. Detox, retox, detox, retox. This pattern felt familiar. I was desperate to find the thing that would work.

I was forced to tell a friend I was struggling with food when I couldn't choose anything from the menu at an all-day brunch cafe. 'I'm hungry all the time,' I told her, 'but I can't digest anything without it hurting.'

'What do you like eating?' she asked.

'I don't remember,' I said.

'This,' I said, gesturing to my plate of tofu, avocado and vegetables when it had arrived.

'Can you just eat a little and stop when you're full?'

'You're telling me to eat intuitively like a normal person,' I snapped. 'I'm never going to be a normal person.'

I disappeared for several months after that, refusing to see friends, and trying to sort myself out. I made meal plans and rules and then failed to stick to them. I felt like I needed rehab but I didn't have the money. At the same time, I didn't want to be told what to do. Having meals monitored, locks on the outside of toilet doors, a ban on exercise – as I'm told goes on in these places – filled me with dread.

In the past staying active, practising yoga daily, seeing friends was the most reliable way for me to stay well, but something wasn't quite working this time. My body had changed, many postures had become uncomfortable to do, and I felt weak physically and emotionally but desperate not to lose my faith in the practice again.

I was working full-time again as a campaigns manager at a charity for a few months. I wasn't teaching yoga. I was still throwing up. One night, I blurted out what had been going on to Stuart in a restaurant. He had never understood my eating problems, so it felt like a foolish move. But he listened to everything that came pouring out of me as I explained why my stomach was so sore, which was why I couldn't finish the masala dosa in front of me.

That night was a turning point. Stuart came to see me every evening for a few weeks to eat with me. It had been his suggestion and I wasn't happy about it because I felt like I was giving up control of my own recovery. But I knew I wouldn't be able to do this alone and I was going to throw everything at it if I was going to be in with a chance of changing anything. I did my best to trust the process. Sometimes Stuart and I would go to restaurants and other times I would prepare a meal in boxes that we would eat in a park and then practise a walking or sitting meditation together until the discomfort in my stomach had passed. It seemed like an extreme measure, but I had no other solutions. Eating with Stuart was our way of trying to recreate what I had lost after my break-up – having a person to share a meal with and therefore a reason to eat. It was a painful process at first and I slipped many times, but slowly, as I did with drinking one day at a time, I was able to eat by myself again without being sick. I was terrified of losing my grip on my practice during what felt like a delicate and transformative time yet again, so I reached out to a yoga teacher friend who had invited me to attend her Mysore classes free of charge and I had never taken her up on it. I started attending them every day and practised at the back of the room. I didn't want any attention. I just needed somewhere to feel safe, to practise in my own way alongside others and to feel less alone.

As part of this period of healing I started teaching yoga again – only once a week at a studio where I felt safe and welcome, because imposter syndrome had crept back in. I questioned whether I was wrong to accept the class given that my demons had come back. I was also worried I might not be well enough to take care of others when I was having to learn how to do it for myself again. I ignored those thoughts and did it anyway. All I could do was turn up, share the practice I knew and hope those who came felt that it was coming from a genuine place.

My class became popular very quickly, which was a huge surprise to me because there was no music and I was teaching Ashtanga, albeit in an adapted way. I started to love teach-ing it and, because I wasn't running around on trains and buses teaching as much as I did before, I looked forward to it each week. And because I knew yoga wasn't ever going to be a career for me, I wasn't doing it for the money this time.

I had found a place to teach in a way I believed in from outside the yoga scene that I had never fitted into. Now I didn't have to. I loved that we practised strong and had a good time doing it. I loved seeing it work for people and that they came back even more. I didn't know that would happen but I was so grateful it did. I discovered that teaching again was helping me in an unexpected way too. It reminded me how crucial my own practice is to me. In this way teaching and taking care of others reminded me to keep taking care of myself.

CHAPTER 11

Fuck Yoga (or Is Yoga Fucked?)

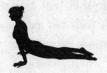

That time of healing and turning inwards as I dealt with disordered eating again felt like one of the most honest periods of my life. I had to admit that I needed to step back into recovery. It was frustrating at first because my life had become unmanageable like it hadn't been since I stopped drinking. My relapse taught me that bulimia and body dysmorphia might be things I have to keep at bay and learn to live with. This was a difficult thing to make peace with at first because I wished I wasn't like this, but it forced me to confront parts of myself that I had overlooked before – namely my fear of abandonment. Losing James showed me that. It also revealed how much a fear of loss was wrapped up in my relationship with love. I knew I was going to have to work through this stuff once and for all. My yoga practice supported me again as I navigated through and I was glad I didn't let it slide this time.

That experience reminded me why I have an endless curiosity and enthusiasm for seeing yoga help others and why it is often the thing people turn to in times of struggle – often for the first time. I love hearing about people getting into yoga. I genuinely do, because I believe in this practice. It's because of this I was drawn to work with outliers, like those teenage boys and the mothers at the first charity class I ever taught. I'm passionate about the practice being made available for those who might not be able to access it through mainstream classes either due to cost, because what's on offer isn't accessible to their emotional and physical needs, or because they don't feel they belong there. I want to see it made available for more people because yoga is a powerful practice that works.

Most people come to yoga because they want to change something. To fix an injury perhaps or other health benefits and a sense of calm – that's why my mum took me, after all. But there's something amiss when marketing campaigns focus merely on the physical part of what yoga can do. This is the main narrative that surrounds yoga as a wellness product to make our lives better. I've found this confusing to make sense of because yoga does make me feel well but not in a clean-eating, scented candles way. That's part of the problem and why I think it's high time the billion-dollar wellness industry takes a hard look at itself. This means businesses, teachers and practitioners taking responsibility and engaging in what might be uncomfortable conversations to examine their part in the current state of play with regards to yoga. I'm not going back on what I've said about it being perfectly acceptable to practise yoga purely for its physical benefits alone, but I think that is coming at a cost given the scale of its appeal.

I noticed this Yoga for a Healthier Lifestyle promotion for the first time one September, which is National Yoga Month in the US. It was introduced by the Department of Health and Human Services in 2008 to educate the nation about the physical benefits of yoga and to inspire a healthy lifestyle. I watched as thousands of yoga fans, fitness professionals and activewear ambassadors took to Instagram to post (and pose) for pictures of themselves performing yoga postures. Sure, many of the posts included captions about how yoga had changed their lives, cultivated self-acceptance, and made life more bearable. I can't argue with that; the same has been true for me. But there was no mention in the Department's campaign of the spiritual practice for self-inquiry that yoga was intended for. It was almost as if people went out of their way to purposely ignore that part of yoga because it suited them. It's faulty messaging like this that perpetuates the wellness industry's idea of what yoga is (and isn't). Given that yoga is an ancient practice that has evolved from a country with a bloody history involving colonization, we should all do better to treat its traditions with more respect.

For this reason, I believe it's important to move away from 'awareness' of a healthy lifestyle towards looking at yoga practice as a whole, acknowledging where it came from, what it was meant for, and inviting practitioners to think about why we spend all that time making those crazy shapes.

Yoga fails to be about wellness or well-being when a practice designed for one thing is being distorted for another. This is what erasure of a culture and specifically cultural appropriation looks like in action. I know I'm not alone in my concerns around cultural appropriation and yoga. When I found my voice through writing about it on social media I discovered others like myself who are using their platforms to change what's happened to yoga too. There are powerful voices in yoga spaces all over the world calling to decolonize yoga and make it more accessible to people of colour. These form part of the important conversations that are happening around yoga and what should happen next. The idea of decolonizing yoga isn't something I've ever felt strongly aligned with even though I understand the sentiment behind it. The word 'decolonize' just doesn't chime with me (even if that's what happened to yoga). I don't think detangling yoga from all traces of Western influence is going to solve the modern yoga problem. Also, South Asia was invaded so many times by different civilizations in the past that it would be impossible to completely distil yoga back to whatever it once was in the beginning. I'm less interested in reclaiming or taking yoga back. I'm more motivated by seeing the practice made accessible for more people who the wellness industry ignores. This is why my call in this book is for a revolution, a fresh take on things. Rather than centring the politics of yoga around the problems of colonization, I think it's more important to look to solutions and how yoga fits in with modern life.

Part of the trouble with yoga in the Western world is that it's become a bit like chicken tikka masala (a popular dish in the UK). Masquerading as something it's not. Neither yoga nor chicken tikka masala is authentically Indian, and yet both pretend to be. Yoga started in ancient India. Chicken tikka masala, on the other hand, was born in a kitchen thousands of miles from the subcontinent. But how it came about remains unclear. Wikipedia will tell you that 'ethnic food historians' believe it was put together by Bengali chefs in Britain, trying to find a way to satisfy English palates. Another explanation credits Pakistani chef Ali Ahmed Aslam, proprietor of the Shish Mahal restaurant in the west end of Glasgow. In 2013, his son Asif Ali told the story to the BBC's Hairy Bikers' TV cookery programme of the curry's invention in 1971 (nine years before I was born). Aslam told the BBC programme: 'A bus driver coming off shift came in and ordered a chicken curry. He sent it back to the waiter, saying it's dry. At the time, Dad had an ulcer and was enjoying a plate of tomato soup. So he said why not put some tomato soup into the curry with some spices. They sent it back to the table and the bus driver absolutely loved it. He and his friends came back again and again and we put it on the menu.'

Both of these sound like plausible stories. This isn't something my mum ever cooked at home, and neither did my grandmother before her. Go to India and I suspect you won't find it either. I don't eat meat, but I've never seen it on menus on my travels. I can't be sure because I'm not a historian but a lot of meat dishes you've eaten in curry houses across the UK might actually be Pakistani (a very meaty nation) or a hangover from the Mughal Empire, given that devout Hindus are vegetarian. It doesn't really matter, but if we're going to think about authenticity for a moment, your favourite thing on that takeaway menu in the kitchen drawer could be an invented variant of any number of South Asian dishes. I tell you this not to digress way off topic but to show you a bit about how cultural appropriation works. The difference is that this dish was invented by a South Asian. So the result isn't as problematic as an outsider coming along and distorting the original object beyond recognition. Yoga, on the other hand, has been repurposed so much that the new Western version has found its way back to South Asia, where Indians themselves are selling yoga the way foreigners want and expect it to be. This is evidence of how deep the effects of colonialism can go. I've seen this firsthand in tourist hotspots in India. So we're in a complicated yoga-web of affairs.

So how did we end up with these problems? Well, the way yoga teacher training itself is taught is a big issue. I realize that I might have made it sound like the life of a yoga teacher is hard work. It is in London because it's tough getting hired, the wages are poor and there are just too many teachers. Becoming a teacher, however, is really easy – if you've got the money to pay for it. It's worth pointing out that the three-month course I did in India wasn't accredited by a Western body so when I went for jobs, employers only paid attention to the one I did in London. It took almost a year to do, but there is training that takes much less time. The yoga industry is riddled with problems and a huge one is thirty-day teacher training courses, which are churning out teachers who I'm afraid to say are unlikely to be skilled enough or equipped to teach.

I just can't believe that it's feasible to become a yoga teacher in a month and I know many long-time yoga teachers who agree. Even worse, there are courses that are entirely online so you don't even come face to face in person with your tutor. This vastly undervalues what it means to be a yoga teacher, and I know lots of teachers who are frustrated with the industry as much as I am – in part because of this crash-course training approach. There are so many body-work professions – massage, osteopathy, acupuncture – that take years to train for, and talking therapy training takes a long time too. If you're going to yoga classes I would scrutinize the background of teachers you're dealing with. I'm happy to talk about my credentials to anyone who asks, because I've done the training and earned the certificates but – more importantly – I've lived a complex life with this practice. This training boom shows us that yoga has been spectacularly hijacked by media, advertising and big business because teacher training courses are a big moneymaker. And yoga teachers are part of the problem because we form part of the industry and have a responsibility to uphold the integrity of the spiritual practice that is yoga.

I met someone who did a month-long teacher training with a wildly popular company in London alongside thirty other people. There were twelve of us on my London course so we had a lot of contact time and discussion with the tutors and I'm still in touch with both of them. But this new teacher who did the course with thirty others described the experience to me as life-changing. And it got me thinking: I paid £3,000 for my training (in instalments) and if there are thirty people on this training and everyone's paying what I did – that's a lot of money. And a hell of a lot of aspiring teachers in want of jobs.

If you're a regular at yoga classes, you might be familiar with the way teachers are certified by the number of hours they have undergone during training. Teachers often put this information on their websites and social media bios such as 200 or 500 hours RYT, which means Registered Yoga Teacher, and SYT means Senior Yoga Teacher. I used these on my CV when I was going for jobs, because employers want to see them. I don't use them any more. This is why I have a problem with the certification structure: I've been practising since I was a teenager – not with as much depth as I do now, of course – but employers never seemed interested in that. They only wanted to know where I trained, who I've taught and possibly how fancy my leggings were (which is why I spent all that cash on that new wardrobe at the beginning).

From what I've seen of a lot of fresh-out-of-yoga-school teachers I met when I worked at the yoga studio, and from some of the bios I've read on schedules, new yoga teachers haven't always practised for very long before they start teaching. In my opinion we should be doing several years of solid practise before teaching anyone, because I really believe length of time with yoga equates to depth of knowledge and a broader experience. I see the teaching as an extension of your own self-inquiry by way of passing on and sharing your own discoveries. How can you do that if you don't spend a bit of time on it before you start saying 'Hey everyone, this is what I've learnt and this is what it means to me'? There shouldn't be any shortcuts.

So what exactly is the problem? Let's take a closer look as I try to make sense of what's going on.

The Unbearable Whiteness of Yoga

There is clearly a whiteness problem within yoga. I say problem because there's a dominance of white people involved whether it's through teaching, practising or owning yoga-related businesses. Why is that? Looked at one way, perhaps it's middle-class white people who need yoga most. If these people are working stressful jobs or have other personal struggles and need a spiritual purpose, yoga could offer that to them. Or looked at another way, maybe most people teaching yoga, practising it or opening studios are in greater positions of privilege with more money and resources to get involved. But I know from my work in leisure centres and teaching vulnerable groups through my outreach work as well as people of colour who have contacted me to teach them online that there's clearly an interest in yoga across a broader demographic than simply white people who have the money for expensive classes.

The trouble with people going to mainstream classes is if they're not being taught to observe yoga holistically by today's teachers, then they're not going to go very far with it. A yoga teacher friend (who also happens to be white) had been thinking about how to make yoga more appealing to people of colour. She told me that she contacted a London studio owner to say she was disappointed about the lack of diversity among teachers at that particular business, which was in an area with a large number of African and Caribbean residents. This annoyed the owner, who then posted screenshots of their private emails to Facebook, saying that she felt attacked. She also went on to say she wasn't going to hire non-white teachers to tick boxes. Sadly, from what I've been told by many other teachers who have tried to bring about change in their communities, this is a common response and also an example of white fragility.

I also saw these issues play out firsthand in my job at the yoga studio. Shortly before I quit, the owners booked a workshop with a marketing agency to look at how they could appeal to a more diverse crowd. It was the owners' attempt to distance themselves from the yoga clichés they had perhaps auto-piloted into (but were at least aware of). I left before the session took place. I sometimes wonder how they're getting on with those plans to diversify because the front of house staff was mostly made up of white women when I worked there. I desperately wanted to get more people of colour in but was only given two weeks to build my team and didn't succeed. From what I saw when I worked at the yoga studio, many people of colour attending were going to classes run by Black and Asian teachers. This reveals that representation matters and makes a difference. But I still don't think it's enough. These teachers have a lot to offer and if they're helping people come to yoga who otherwise might not, I'm happy. But these teachers of colour are still working within a flawed industry so are operating within a system that is ultimately oppressive to others like themselves. This gives me the feeling that the only real solution to yoga's problems is a massive shake-up, a revolution – not merely integration.

I was inspired by the idea of revolution after listening to Kehinde Andrews, Professor of Black Studies at Birmingham

City University and author of the excellent *Back to Black*,[31] on Russell Brand's *Under the Skin* podcast.[32] He talked about revolution as being the only solution to liberate Black people because: 'You can't trust people in the West who benefit from a system to end that system'. He also explains that 'whiteness is a philosophy that engages Black and Brown people too'. I have experienced this when I've been attacked by yoga teachers of colour on Instagram for things I have written, only for them to praise and uphold the current wellness system with its *Namastay in bed* slogans. Andrews refers to this internalized form of white supremacy as the psychosis of whiteness and references Conservative commentator Candice Owens as an example of what happens – 'we go mad' – when we as people of colour choose to integrate. Owens is best known for her pro-Donald Trump commentary and her criticism of liberal rhetoric regarding structural racism, systemic inequality and the Black Lives Matter movement, which all came as a baffling move in 2017 given that she had been a supporter of these issues just a few years earlier. If whiteness had made Owens go mad, maybe it's what happened to me, too. I certainly felt crazy when I was working at the yoga studio.

I'm glad I left before the marketing workshop took place, which might sound like I don't care. I can tell you that I do care – more than a lot of people. But I got the sense that this workshop was more about making the owners feel better about themselves and be seen to be doing something than actually effecting any change. Plus, I'd seen it happen before. The place I had volunteered at in 2000 expanded to own several studios across London, and hastily changed its marketing materials in the summer of 2018. A post on the company's social media accounts had called for people to be part of a new campaign they planned to run, featuring those they described as 'people of colour/fat/thin/disabled/trans/queer – essentially every kind of body out there'. I went along to the photoshoot out of curiosity and looked on as an art director and cameraman appeared to identify anyone who looked the part to zoom in on for the promotional video they were filming. I'm talking about Afro hair, tattoos, piercings, people of colour, or anyone who could pass as not-white, and so on. We were led by a teacher who was there to guide us to make it look like we were doing a yoga class.

Ironically, it seemed that some people at the shoot didn't even practise at this swanky brand's chain of studios. I got chatting to one of them, an Indian man wearing billowing trousers and an admirable twirling moustache. He told me that he saw a post about the shoot on Facebook and thought it looked fun. It was his first time at the studio and he in fact attended yoga classes at a David Lloyd gym. I understand that it's important for yoga business owners to look like they're finally doing something by organizing workshops or arranging a social media marketing campaign. It's well meaning but the intention behind these moves remains questionable. Surely in this day and age we want to see a range of diversity in yoga across as many spectrums as possible, but changing the imagery of websites to include visuals of different-looking people while a good move, only addresses the surface of the yoga problem. It is a tokenism that might even make things worse in the long run.

In the end, the workshop and the photoshoot just made me feel incredulous that diversity hadn't been a priority in yoga a long time ago and angry at myself that I'd thought it had been a good idea to go. It's worth saying that the founder of this same studio sent a lengthy newsletter out after George Floyd was murdered by police in the US in May 2020. He wrote a beautifully written, heartfelt letter of apology for overlooking accessibility and diversity in the twenty years since the company opened their first studio. I read his carefully worded piece and really wanted to believe he understood. But I remembered hearing him in an online recording of a talk discussing diversity in yoga hosted by his own company, suggesting that he didn't think it was right to put someone behind the front desk for the 'sake of it' or the 'wrong reasons'. In fairness, when responding to a question from the audience he did go on to say: 'I genuinely would like to have more representatives of our society at our front desk so that people felt more comfortable . . . and if you could tell us how to do that more, I'd like to know.' I finished listening to the recording shaking my head because I find it incredibly bemusing that white people always seem to need advice – often from people of colour – on how to make their workforces more diverse. Why is it so hard to do? Also, diversity isn't just about skin colour, which is the first thing – particularly since George Floyd – that businesses have rightfully felt pressured to acknowledge. Forgive me for being obsessed with class and life experience but they are so important. I am living proof, because I worked at a yoga studio where my being there might have helped represent a part of the community – but I still felt like the odd one out because I was surrounded by people who had different life experiences and lifestyles to me. I'll never stop feeling working class because of where I've come from and the experiences I've had. I have more privileges than I've had in the past but I haven't forgotten how hard it was to get here, and I know when I'm in spaces that don't have people like me in mind.

The *British Medical Journal* published a survey[33] in October 2020 called 'Yoga practice in the UK: a cross-sectional survey of motivation, health benefits and behaviours'. Of the 2,635 people who responded, only 2,434 people met the inclusion criteria. Of the 2,434 respondents 69.3 per cent said they had experienced positive lifestyle changes as a result of their yoga practice. The statistics for other improvements they saw are as follows:

- Improved physical health (88 per cent)
- Mental health (86.2 per cent)
- Stress levels (82.6 per cent)
- Strength (87.1 per cent) and flexibility (91.6 per cent)
- Sleep improvement (57.4 per cent)

Well, we knew that already, was my first thought as I read through the whole survey that just served to provide numbers for what seemed obvious. My second thought was: *who took part?* So here you go, this is a direct paragraph from the published survey:

> *The majority of respondents were women, white, well educated, with a wide age range (18–92). Participants rated themselves as above average in terms of subjective social status. All areas of the UK were represented although London and the south-east of England were most prevalent. Forty per cent of the sample were yoga teachers.*

This tells us that the survey was mainly undertaken by affluent white women, of whom just under half were yoga teachers. This also shows us that we're only hearing from one kind of person, and seems to imply that no one else is interested in yoga. Something's not right, is it?

I'll do my best to dig into some of it here. Grab yourself a masala chai and let's take a look at what the new yoga has become in more detail.

Yoga is White-washed

When you're a person of colour, you notice that most people going to yoga classes are white. But there's not a lot you can do, so you ignore it and get on with your practice. That's what I've always done. Diversity is deeply absent in most yoga classes, and I'm not sure why. It's always appeared that way for me, since I went to my first class in 1996. It didn't bother me back then but I was just at the start of my journey and yoga wasn't as big as it is today. So why are there so few people of colour in yoga classes? It could be that people of colour are more likely to follow a religion or have had a background involving theist teachings that may appear to them to be in conflict with yoga due to its links with Hinduism. The philosophical side of the practice is also geared towards a connection with a higher consciousness, which could sound a lot like God.

The other issue might be that seeing an industry filled with overwhelmingly white teachers and students puts people of colour off. I've received messages from many people who feel this way. Most teachers of classes I've attended in the past have been white. Though I noticed this – because when you're a person of colour you *always* notice this – it didn't affect me because I was wrapped up in my own practice. That is, until I started teaching. This meant that I was often the only person of colour in the room and it felt strange in a teaching role. I was thrilled whenever a non-white person came through the door. Just because you've spent your life being in a minority and got used to it, doesn't mean you like it.

As already mentioned in chapter 8, leisure centre classes were a bit more ethnically mixed than classes in yoga studios, in my experience, which was revealing from an economic point of view. People of colour are often statistically poorer than their white neighbours, so if they're into yoga they might be in with a chance of affording it at their local leisure centre. It's tough teaching in leisure centres – there aren't any fancy mats or props to assist, but I found it deeply rewarding. I've not come face to face with more injuries, health conditions, different body types, ages or genders than I did in those places, and as a result I learnt more about teaching there than any-where else. If you can hack it as a teacher in a leisure centre, I'm convinced you can teach anywhere. It's proper graft work and more teachers could do with working there. Yet some teachers are unaware that yoga is even offered there.

'Do people really still go to the gym for yoga?' asked an Ashtanga teacher whose dogmatic vibe I didn't like and whose poorly attended class I covered once in her absence. I'd been telling her about my work in leisure centres.

'Yeah – the classes I teach there are always packed,' I said.

'That's interesting. I don't know if yoga belongs in gyms though,' she said.

The diversity of income, body shape, ability and so on in leisure centres reminds you about service: you're working in an actual community. Yoga should be available for anyone who wants it and, when it's affordable, it can be.

As I've said, lack of diversity was also common at auditions. A friend I met on the 2016 teacher training in London thought this could work in my favour.

'Don't you find that you're at an advantage over others?' she asked as we walked towards the East London community centre where I taught.

'Why, because I look Indian?' I asked.

'Yeah, I would have thought people feel they're getting something more authentic with you,' she said.

'But I'm not Indian,' I said.

'They don't know that,' she told me.

'But it's not like I'm trying to sell myself as a yoga expert or claim I know more about it than anyone else,' I said.

'Yeah, but you've practised for a long time.' My friend had a point.

'Doesn't make a difference. I don't think anyone even notices that I'm Asian,' I said. 'My skin colour is definitely not doing me any favours.'

Yoga is Commercialized

And incredibly so. Yoga might save your mind, body and spirit but not until it's taken all your money. It's become exclusive, elitist and, at anywhere up to £20 a class, expensive. Buying a class pack or monthly pass can set you back over £150 depending on where you're going. An annual membership would be well over £1,000 and you'd have to go to a lot of classes to make it worth it. Despite this, teachers' pay remains low. This kind of capitalism and lack of regard for teachers' welfare is just plain wrong, never mind being at odds with the ethics of yoga – which it doesn't sit well with either.

Interestingly, it seems the bigger the yoga business, the lower the pay – not always, but when I asked around teachers I know who teach at hugely expensive and successful studios they didn't seem to be earning a whole lot more than me. This is the opposite of how things work in the corporate world, where you're likely to be paid more when working at a big company and less if you were at a start-up. I found that the owners of independent studios I worked at were trying to offer a pay structure that gave teachers a better deal. The money wasn't great but it isn't great anywhere. Yet I didn't feel ripped off at the independents, and it made the teaching experience so much more enjoyable.

Generally, teachers are paid between £20 and £35 an hour, which usually goes up if the class is longer. This is not a lot of money. The fees are along these lines in leisure centres – I got £27.69 as a casual staff member. Senior teachers can command more, but length of teaching experience doesn't always translate into high quality, from what I've seen. Of course, it's important but, as you know from the horror stories of some so-called senior teachers I shared in chapter 6, a teacher's own personal practice and conduct in life is far more important than the number of certificates they hold or hours they've taught.

A studio receptionist told me that a big studio in London hires people based on their social media following. 'I'm never going to be working there,' I had joked with her. I understand that these celebrity teachers pull in the numbers to fill classes, and businesses need to stay afloat, but there's an economic problem here. It leads to classes becoming exclusive because they're not affordable and means that the hiring process isn't democratic and based on actual merit. I feel like it also creates a divide, where the celebrity teacher is the shining light and the underlings are the students who flock to the classes, which creates a space for the ego to move into. We don't want to be massaging the ego. Yoga is there to help us to observe the ego and keep it in its place. It can encourage us to become more self-aware and less self-centred.

Some yoga studios offer teachers a basic fee, which goes up incrementally depending on how many people come to the class. Others offer a £10 bonus or similar if you hit twenty students but that's not guaranteed, particularly if you're a cover teacher. Classes with a cover teacher might dissuade regulars, who won't always come if their usual guru isn't available.

Annoyingly, I once covered a class with nineteen students. There's also another pay structure where a studio pays £25 and then £1 per person who turns up. This works out brilliantly in financial terms if lots of people come, but it's a gamble.

For workplace and private sessions, I've been paid between £40 and £60 a session. This might sound like a lot for an hour's work but, once you factor in travel cost and the time it takes to get there and back, the money quickly starts to dwindle. Running around on public transport between classes is exhausting too – particularly in London. I spent most of my teaching days on trains in the past but it was hard to turn work down because I never had enough money. On the hottest day of the year in summer 2019, I overdid it, and taught four classes in a single day. This isn't unusual for some teachers, but these were all over the city in central, North, East and South London. The first one was at 8 a.m.; I got home from the last one at 10 p.m. and made £140. I enjoyed the work, and everyone gave me wonderful feedback so it kept me going back, but it burnt me out in the end. Teaching is not a lucrative life. Steps have been taken to address the wage issue, with a teachers' union launched in New York in the summer of 2019, and the Yoga Teacher's Union that Norman talked to me about established in the UK in October 2020.

I've spent a hell of a lot of money on yoga over the twenty-odd years I've been going to classes. Even when the cost bothered me, I coughed up and – lucky me – I could just about afford it. Ironically it got harder to afford when I started teaching, because I didn't earn enough to justify the spend. The priciness of yoga and the training to teach, suggests that wellness is a privilege, and it shouldn't be. Yoga and #selfcare can be yours for the taking, but only if you can pay for it, it seems. I understand that people need to make money to keep their yoga businesses going, but there's a balance to be struck. When people complained about the cramped conditions due to the number of mats in the studios at the place I worked, the owners said they'd lose several thousand pounds per year if they removed any. It didn't matter that customers told me they couldn't move freely when classes were fully booked.

I got some £40-an-hour work through a Deliveroo-like app offering private teaching. This business charged customers £69 so the mark-up on what they pocketed themselves was high. Customers could book a session through the app, and a yogi would be 'delivered' to their door, not unlike pizza. It turned out to be a stressful way to work because you marked yourself as available on the app and then had to wait – for weeks at a time, in my case – to see if anyone booked. This isn't ideal for an anxious person like me because you couldn't make any personal plans and were kind of on call, waiting for work that didn't always come. I lugged a 2kg, eco-friendly mat, yoga blocks and blanket to East Finchley for my debut booking on a Saturday night. On the Northern Line journey home, I realized that I myself had become commercialized. I was now the commodity bearing yogic gifts, and it didn't feel good. I dropped that job after a few months.

My final booking came when I was sitting on a park bench, recalibrating myself after therapy. I did a double-take because I recognized the surname of a famously wealthy family. I wore my smartest leggings and best hoodie for the appointment for which the client was fifteen minutes late. I was blithe and relaxed about the experience because I'm generally not fazed when faced with staggering privilege, but I was fascinated by what I might see inside her home (she had three Francis Bacon paintings in the living room). She was pleasant, but also guarded and kept repeating 'thank you so much' after almost every instruction in that way I imagine people do when everything's always been done for them. I briefly fantasized about teaching her every day, ending in us becoming best friends and never having any money worries again. But of course life doesn't go like that, and as I walked back to the Tube station I felt that angry knot that lives in my stomach come back because, millionaire client or not, I would still only get paid £40. I resigned because the pay wasn't sustainable and I decided it wasn't worth sticking around just to be part of a social experiment.

Yoga-inflationary pressures mean that yoga training is expensive too. One of the big reasons I didn't undertake yoga teacher training for so long was because I didn't have a spare £3,000 to pay for it. I did the course over a series of weekends while I had a full-time communications job. It's the only way I could have found the time and money to do it. I wouldn't have been able to take a month or six weeks out of my life to go to Costa Rica or Thailand for intensive training and return to work. As I previously mentioned, when training courses cost as much as they do and are attended by thirty-odd people, some people are certainly making money out of yoga. But I have definitely not been one of them.

Yoga is Trendy

To the point of being – or perhaps already far beyond – clichéd. There are trappings: plant-based diets, free-spirited good vibes only, mesh-leggings; and it often feels like yoga today is a parody or has somewhere down the line become a victim of itself. You know a culture is in trouble when it's been boiled down to a handful of clichés that obscure or pervert what it was actually meant to be about. If you suddenly arrived from

Mars, you'd be forgiven for thinking that there seems to be a type of person who goes to yoga classes – frequently characterized as smug and pleased with themselves, often middle class, probably a cisgender woman, naturally flexible, well off, often blonde, slim-limbed, and white.

I'm generalizing, of course, but there's some truth in this characterization. These people go to yoga brunch workshops and buy gut-nourishing smoothies on the way out. They've started adding turmeric to everything they eat because of its healing properties, while non-vegans might be experimenting with ghee. Among other effects, this leads to people like me with South Asian heritage, who have spent a lifetime eating smelly dishes with these ingredients, getting an uncomfortable sense of what it feels like when your culture's suddenly on trend. Getting a tattoo also seems to be popular, preferably featuring a Hindu god or Sanskrit writing no one can read. Or perhaps a design that resembles a henna pattern. Proudly telling everyone you've got a 'plant-based' diet is standard especially on social media profiles. Being vegan is, of course, good for the earth and many have turned to this lifestyle due to our planet's climate emergency, but at times it seems as though it's also become a status symbol. As does sporting branded activewear, buying the latest props, water bottles, and hot-off-the-shelf mats you never knew you needed. It's not just women, of course: broga (yoga and fitness for blokes) and the growth in yoga wear labels for men suggest dudes are just as prey to the clichés as women.

Yoga is now a fixture of flat-white-drinking, sourdough-munching, craft-beer-supping hipsterdom. If you live in a gentrifying urban area – watch out, there'll be a yoga studio there soon (if there isn't already). Many of these features of modern yoga are observable in real life, but for the real tick there's social media, where the output inevitably involves these crop-topped or bare-chested practitioners filming themselves doing their morning practice. Or getting someone else to snap them performing advanced Asanas – usually with hands on floor and legs in the air. Otherwise, it might be moody skies accompanied by life-affirming quotes from the widely lauded Persian poet Rumi.

Sadly, there's also a type of person who teaches yoga, judging by what dominates Instagram. These people travel to exotic places and take selfies of themselves drinking from coconuts with the wind in their hair. This might be when they're in India undergoing their 200-hour training to teach. They 'love' India, of course. Even though most of those who go are likely to have spent all their time in a secluded beach resort, meaning they've not experienced the properly exhausting, at times exasperating (especially if you're a woman) and chaotic (albeit mesmerizing) place it can be. If you've never tried to buy a train ticket or taken a long journey on public transport in India, you hand-on-heart haven't seen enough to form an honest opinion.

Yogis also like taking pictures of their avocado on toast and chia seed breakfast bowls, and letting us know that they've 'got 99 problems, but yoga ain't one'. Why? Because they're 'wellness warriors', which means their sweat probably smells of strawberries . . . or patchouli. It makes you wonder what's behind all these trends. To me, it looks like everyone wants to be in an exclusive #liveyourbestlife gang.

In some ways, fair enough. The way it's told culturally, yoga is now about wellness. And in a way this isn't so far from the truth. One of the fundamentals of yoga is about behaving well towards oneself and the world. This is laid out in the Eight Limbs of Yoga (see page 82), which are less about being 'well' than something much deeper: a way of living. But also, all that permanently positive stuff we see so much of on social media doesn't resonate for me. Given the life I've had, I'm happy to say I'm done with the misery trap, but I also think owning one's pain and mishaps and being real about it can be what becomes the true beauty of life in the end. It's the pain that often teaches us about what's really important, rather than pretending everything's beautiful and jolly all the time.

In other words, real yoga is a serious practice, and nothing to do with smoothies or branded leggings on social media. But this formal way of working with yoga isn't quite what we've ended up with. It's been pulled up from its roots, and this new yoga appears to have grown in its place as one of the most coveted ways to reach your #lifegoals by coolhunters in search of the latest health trend. It's a way to get fit and somehow be a better person, because there's a spiritual element in there somewhere. Handy for those with an 'I'm not religious but I'm spiritual' outlook too.

While we're here, shamanic healing, gong baths, cacao ceremonies, sound therapy and reiki are other popular wellness clichés too, since many yoga teachers offer them as part of their work. They're all wonderful things – some of which I've personally enjoyed trying out – but each extend from different cultures. So it's bemusing to me that they're frequently offered as part of the same package. They've got nothing to do with yoga.

Yoga Is Not an Addiction

Yoga sometimes thinks it's an addiction. It isn't. Added to the clichés above, there's a language that yoga borrows from elsewhere – namely addiction recovery. Inhabitants of the wellness world often declare themselves (on social media, at least) to be a 'yoga junkie' or 'handstand addict'. I met a new-ish yoga teacher who came to a class I taught and told me that she was 'addicted' to her practice. Language is important. If you're not an actual addict or in recovery from addiction, you shouldn't make fun of those who are or have been. These aren't your words to own.

One summer when I was still living with James, we noticed drug dealing in our street. It wouldn't have troubled me if it was cannabis, but we could tell it was harder stuff. We'd see the customers and they weren't well. I suspect the police knew what was going on but the dealers were clever and knew how to hide. I mention this because I'd dropped into a class with a popular teacher who described a posture we were doing as 'like another pose you might know . . . but on crack'. A friend told me this teacher said that kind of thing all the time. Another teacher mentioned that this same yogi was seen snorting cocaine at the studio's Christmas party. I've talked about this before (see page 136) but here's another reason for not putting your teacher on a pedestal.

I've never taken crack, but I've seen and know what hard drugs can do. So when I meet people who say they're addicted to their yoga practice, or I see posts on social media where people use words like addict and junkie or marketing slogans like 'support your local endorphin dealer' used flippantly, I feel it isn't right. Many people come to yoga when they're dealing with mental struggles and/or illness. For that reason, yoga should strive to be a neutral space. Many of us are doing it to learn about ourselves and deepen connection to ourselves. Addiction and its associated trauma is no joke. So yoga and the people who do it should stop pretending it is.

Yoga is Bastardized

I'm not against innovation, but let's take a moment to think about Voga (some kind of Madonna-inspired fitness meets voguing disaster offered in the UK), Beer and Wine yoga, Gin and Yin yoga, Puppy yoga, Hip Hop and Spliff yoga (in California). There are also new variants that combine yoga with other movement forms and sports aimed at sculpting, lifting, tightening and strengthening our bodies because yoga as it was intended clearly isn't enough. I'm talking about yoga and martial arts, boxing and yoga, weight-lifting and yoga, HIIT to Savasana. These things actually exist.

Alco-yoga seems particularly strange, considering that yoga is about getting in touch with yourself, not getting out of your head. So the claim that 'a small amount of alcohol' might help to facilitate 'relaxation into the poses' on an advert for such an event that I spotted seemed confusing. It's not 'inclusive' for people who don't want to drink. In fairness, the gin wasn't compulsory, but getting tipsy feels like it defeats the object of becoming more mentally clarified when practising yoga.

The most popular classes in the West tend to be Vinyasa Flow or some other 'flow' derivative that tells you to 'expect to get a sweat on'. The flow refers to the movements in between the poses and the job is to observe the breath on the way to the next posture. But too often I've seen that transitions get decorated and garnished, making way for things like three-legged dogs or fussy plank poses with one foot stacked on the other on the way down. In other scenarios I've seen people flinging themselves through the poses so that it's almost as if they're dancing – and I've seen some teachers presenting yoga to classes as if it is a dance. It's not. The postures exist to serve a purpose: to strengthen and purify the body (in preparation for mediation), but also to discipline and focus our unruly minds. How can you do that when you're trying to get through a complicated sequence? You can't. It's worth saying that some teachers will talk about certain postures like twists being good for detoxing. Nope. My experience of doing twists is that they can be uncomfortable but they're good to do because with practise you find more space in your body and a bigger range of movement. As far as I know, they're not medically proven to detox you any more than juice fasts. And I say this as someone who likes a juice cleanse (even though it's bloody hard to do) for the stillness and quiet it brings to the body. But in my extensive research into the benefits of juice fasting, I've yet to find any solid scientific evidence to back up their cleansing claims even if they do give our digestive system a rest, flood the body with vitamins and help us feel lighter (let's face it, many of us embark on such things expecting life-changing weight loss or to reduce calorie consumption – unless that's just me and the disordered part of my brain talking now).

In my experience, too many classes focus more on the bits in between poses and that means you don't get to stay in the postures long enough to fully experience each shape your body is making. It's important to pause, breathe and stay in the pose, otherwise the muscles don't have a chance to respond. Which means there's no hope of anything changing. And I'm guessing a lot of us go to yoga classes because we want to change something: physically, emotionally, dare I say spiritually. I'm happiest when I'm moving my body, and I've tried lots of movement activities in the past – ecstatic dance, 5Rhythms, gym workouts and free flow movement, for instance. Embodied movement and primal movement are genuinely lovely things but they're not yoga. Yoga probably shouldn't be placed in the middle of a trance party, though given the number of 'yoga raves' I've seen hosted in the last few years, others may disagree.

All of this makes me wonder how much some teachers actually respect yoga when they're so keen on distorting it into something it's not. Mandala, Vinyasa Flow, Prana Flow, Creative Flow, Restorative, Rocket and Budokon are all contemporary remakes of traditional Hatha and Ashtanga yoga (the latter was developed after Hatha and was the original Vinyasa style). The newer incarnations of yoga have been crafted by Westerners for whom the original methods were evidently not good enough. I'm not suggesting all of the new versions of yoga must go in the bin but I do question why we need such a dizzying selection. Yoga in practice is quite simple, and so many different styles make it more complicated than it needs to be.

I've tried most styles at least once, but even I can't keep up. I was once asked to cover a class at a gym and when I requested more information on what was expected, the teacher said 'Strala'. It was the first I'd heard of it. (It combines Tai Chi and yoga, since you ask.) I had to turn that job down. There's also a yoga where goats are set loose to walk around as you practise. It's also not right for yoga to be an exercise class, though of course that's what you'll find in most places, even if you're told you're attending a mind and body class – you're still working out. I'd admit that Acro yoga – where you're suspended in a hammock or supported by a partner while levitating in the air – is fun, but calling it yoga causes problems because the more stuff we call yoga, the harder it becomes to discern what the original purpose of this practice was.

A class shouldn't be deemed better or worse because of its playlist either, but it often is. Teachers are known for their beats when they should be celebrated for their knowledge, personal practice and attention to people attending their classes. I love music and often listen to dancehall, jungle or grime on my way to teach, but music's not meant for inside the class. I used it when people have expected it, but my choices tended towards the minimal, almost imperceptible beats in the background. Of course, music in some cultures is regarded as helping the spiritual process: chanting, for example. When I was growing up, my mum was a fan of Nusrat Fateh Ali Khan, who was a Pakistani singer of Qawwali, which is a form of Sufi Islamic devotional music. I got into it too – the lyrics are poetic and almost always about God. We went to see him perform in London shortly before his death in 1997, and I was entranced by his voice and delivery. The same object of affection in poems by Persian poets Rumi and Hafiz is God too, by the way. They were both Muslim, which is why I find their popularity on yoga teachers' and wellness practitioners' Instagram feeds so amusing. The poets' philosophizing was often devotional, and intended outwards, instead of encouraging us to love ourselves more. In the end, I can see the benefit of music as a therapeutic aid, but a yoga class shouldn't rely on it.

Yoga is Indian

Well, yes it is. But it's not as simple as that, so let's think about this a little more. I know that some people want to claim yoga as Indian and therefore Hindu, and this is a complex issue that I touched on in Chapter 4. It's not helped by the fact that yoga has been used as a political tool by Narendra Modi, India's Prime Minister at the time of writing this book. The International Day of Yoga, for example, established in 2014 at the United Nations General Assembly, was his idea. Every year there are events across India on 21 June to celebrate it, and on social media everyone takes to writing posts about how much they love yoga. For me, this is further proof of how yoga in the West has gone so far in its exoticization of India that it totally disregards what's going on in modern-day Indian politics. It's so hard to watch so I usually turn my phone off and wait until it passes. The trouble for me is that Modi's politics aren't the most harmonious. His time in office has seen the rise of Hindutva, a right-wing, fundamentalist movement that condones the persecution of Muslims – and indeed anyone who isn't Hindu.

There's another ambivalence that I deal with here because I'm of course not actually Indian. In a way it doesn't really matter because I often identify more as Punjabi anyway. Punjab is both India and Pakistan. I've been to the state of Punjab on both sides of the India and Pakistan border. I've met Punjabi Muslims, Hindus and Sikhs and we're all the same in so many ways. It's a cultural thing. Punjabis are stereotyped as being loud and gregarious (maybe annoyingly for some), they are known for being open-hearted, having fun and taking any excuse for a get-together or celebration that itself might be a bit over the top. I'd say there's some truth in the stereotype, at least in my family and Punjabis I've met. That's why I like them!

We have to remember that India was carved up after the British Empire. Lots of yoga teachers talk about India, and yoga as being a sacred practice from that land, which is true but it's also problematic because India used in this way becomes synonymous with the whole of South Asia and doesn't take into account Bangladesh, Nepal, Pakistan and Sri Lanka. The British Empire saw that the subcontinent got chopped into several pieces in 1947 (the partition of India and formation of East and West Pakistan) and 1971 (the creation of Bangladesh, formerly East Pakistan). So many people involved in the business of yoga seem to be ignorant of this fact. That said, I don't believe that South Asians should have a claim over yoga. We're all outsiders to this ancient culture, that's why when we practise yoga, we should do it with integrity and respect.

All the traditions and cultures that were going on in ancient India at the time that yoga emerged between five and ten thousand years ago should be valued and acknowledged because yoga has come from that pre-colonized place. Yoga is Indian, but India was a different place back then, so I tend to think of yoga as a South Asian practice. I realize this might be an unpopular opinion, and it's not my intention to deny yoga its roots, but I do think we need to look at modern politics and acknowledge the traumas that people have gone through in the past. Many of them are still alive, or like me have learnt about what happened because we're descendents of those people. My grandmother (RIP) lived through partition. So while it's great to have studied yogic tradition, Sanskrit and the rest, I believe it's essential to look at modern life. I don't mean just looking at the lives of urban stressed-out Western people who might need yoga, but also being aware of the lives of immigrants in diaspora communities.

I think a lot of yoga problems might be solved and less harm caused by thinking about how South Asians might perceive the state of modern yoga. I think anyone who works with or practises yoga has a duty to learn about the history of where this thing comes from, what the countries of yoga's origin have been through and what the people who are from there have survived. I've learnt about the impact of the past through growing up with South Asian people of all faiths so it didn't take me a lot of effort. I also learnt about it through watching India and Pakistan play cricket as a kid, which always felt like a politically charged match that was about more than just sport. I don't know if this has changed in the game because I don't follow it anymore. It's possibly less loaded on the pitch now because liberal Indians and Pakistanis are not at war, but there is a historical trauma, sometimes anger, since they were pitted against each other because of the British Empire. Know the history – not just of yoga but of the land and of the people.

Yoga is Culturally Appropriated

Appropriation in yoga is the word Namaste on your T-shirt, it's wearing endless Mala beads. It's tattoos of Sanskrit and Hindu gods and pictures of handstands on beaches by bendy almost-always able-bodied people. It's turmeric lattes and fashionable activewear. This is modern yoga – a practice morphed by Western imperialists into a new lifestyle that's way beyond recognition. But it doesn't have to be. It most definitely shouldn't be.

I know cultural appropriation is a confusing and triggering topic for some people, but we won't be able to get away from it until it stops happening. I still get messages from people asking me what the difference is between appropriation and appreciation, despite having talked about the issue for a long time. So for anyone still confused: nuts-and-bolts cultural appropriation is taking a thing out of context and repackaging it as something else that it isn't. Others have contacted me to suggest there's a fine line between appropriation and appreciation, but I don't see it. Or if there is a line, I see it get rubbed out a lot by people looking for ways to excuse their behaviour when it suits them.

One could argue that we're all appropriating to some degree because yoga is so old. The appropriation in this case isn't really the issue, but how we practise it, which again brings us back to integrity and respect. I often feel that the people who hate talking about cultural appropriation tend to be those who could do with paying attention to it the most. But let's, for argument's sake, say that there is a fine line because I do spend a great deal of time grappling with this issue myself. I call this being culturally sensitive, and more of us could be better at it. For clarity, there's nothing wrong with cooking South Asian food or wearing a sari to your Indian friend's wedding. Try an Indian accent while ordering a curry, however, and you're on shaky ground. It's racist so obviously don't. As a Pakistani, bindis have never had any significance in my own life so I asked an Indian friend how she felt about white women wearing them at music festivals. She rolled her eyes and said: 'It's annoying but whatevs.' My take on that is that it's probably not the worst thing anyone can do but it's clearly not great either. Taking on a new name and wearing a turban, as a lot of white Kundalini yoga teachers do, feels odd to me even if it's done with an Indian man's blessing, and I'm ambivalent about white people teaching Bollywood dance workshops but I don't know if I'm right to be.

In terms of yoga, of course it's fine to practise and learn from it. It's brilliant and I want you to. I've got mixed feelings about chanting, and if you must do it or teach it, it might be helpful to learn what the words mean and to pronounce them better. It also bugged me for a long time (like at that Starbucks audition) when I found myself in the company of teachers who judged my teaching as below par or frowned at any mention of Ashtanga and then celebrated their own method – usually a sweaty exercise class filled with 'juicy flows' set to a banging playlist with a Namaste thrown in at the end. At the same time, when non-Indian yoga teachers speak wistfully of Mother India, I feel it's misplaced too. I can't tell if it's out of respect or because they wish deep down that they were Indian. If you're not an Indian – by birth, heritage or genes – sorry, but you can't claim India as your mother.

Some people argue that what's happened to yoga is straight-up colonialism, that it's been stolen from India by the West, repackaged and resold for the benefit of Westerners. I agree. But I also think most Indian teachers would have wanted the practice to spread. Many Indian teachers from back in the day travelled abroad themselves in order to do this. Many still do – though now it tends to be more of a 'guru on tour' type of affair, so that their disciples across the world have a chance to practise in the presence of their 'master' – usually alongside hundreds of others. My point is that the problem is not how widespread yoga has become but the extent to which yoga is being taken and divorced from its roots.

Younger and more contemporary South Asian teachers are themselves working within the wellness industry that exists today too, so how bad can the problem be, you ask? Well, just because Indian teachers or teachers of colour have found a place to integrate within the wellness industry, or have perhaps reconciled the way that it operates, doesn't make it right. This is why I talk so much about representation not being enough. We don't get away with being part of the system because we're people of colour. Not all people of colour hold the same political views or outlooks on life. I've met many I strongly disagree with, which is proof that our skin colour does not always unite us. The only way I've made peace with teaching yoga is by talking openly about what I see as having gone wrong. I can't be part of the solution while I'm in the problem. I'm still an outlier outside the mainstream and I feel I am in a better position to help improve things from over here. It's my hope that this book can form part of my contribution.

In an episode of his eponymous podcast,[34] Adam Buxton interviewed the Jamaican novelist Marlon James, who had plenty of excellent things to say about race politics. I agreed with everything he said, but he made a particular point about cultural appropriation. There's appropriation and then there's taking something from a culture and pretending you came up with it yourself. He cited Peter Gabriel as a great example of borrowing from different cultures but also crediting and supporting artists from those cultures, also known as amplifying underrepresented voices. Perhaps the armies of new teachers entering the yoga field should ask, 'What would Peter Gabriel do?'

Here's a story about something Gabriel wouldn't do. A yoga teacher mate of mine told me she was upset about having seen the Hindu god Ganesh reimagined on a new T-shirt design from an activewear brand. The elephant god, who is believed to be the 'remover of obstacles', is usually seen holding several objects – all of which have significant symbolic meaning. Yet there he was (with several more arms than his usual four), holding what looked like the following amid several other unidentifiable icons:

a happy-face emoji (or was that an ecstasy tablet?)

a bottle (of kombucha? Or was it booze?)

the two standard male and female gender signs (and no sight of trans and non-binary symbols).

The designer may as well have shoved a pack of ciggies (or a spliff?) into Ganesh's hands while they were at it. I wasn't personally offended when I saw it, because I'm not Hindu. However, I could see that it was wrong, and Hindus would be justified if they took offence.

What Namaste Actually Means

This is a good opportunity to talk about the word Namaste. You'll hear it on the lips of a yoga teacher near you. You might have heard a teacher say it at the end of class, meaning you can go home now. It's on activewear, all over social media and dropped into yoga and wellness newsletters. I've written and talked about the misuse of this word on Instagram and on podcasts many times, and been contacted by dozens of yoga teachers saying they don't say it anymore because of me. This is brilliant. I'm glad my work has had an impact, but I've wondered why they hadn't questioned its relevance earlier and am troubled that it had gone on so long before I came along and switched the lights on. This makes me think it must be coming through teacher trainings, which begs the question: what other misappropriated education are people receiving on their courses?

A US teacher commented on one of my Namaste posts: 'I use the translation of the light within me bows to the light within you, and say that in class followed by Namaste. It's a beautiful sentiment and gives a nod to the Hindu roots of the practice. I don't think all teachers use it in disrespectful or unrelated ways.' Another UK-based teacher asked: 'Do we know how it leaked into yoga?' This is an excellent question and one I can only hypothesize about. It could be that a bunch of Westerners went to India, let's say in the Swinging Sixties, found yoga, then went back home to share it in their communities. So far so good. It could be that they then felt a need to acknowledge yoga's 'Indian-ness' (also a good move) and thought it appropriate to pick an 'exotic' word used in modern India. And years later, it has ended up on T-shirts and in yoga classes. So in a way, Namaste feels a little like an 'I went to India and learnt this word' badge of honour.

The facts
Namaste is a Hindu greeting not an Indian one. This is an important distinction. There are a lot of South Asians in the UK (and the rest of the world) who, like me, aren't Indian. More importantly, there are thousands of people living in

India who aren't Hindu. Namaste has got nothing to do with them – or yoga – which means that the misguided teacher who reached out to me was nodding in the wrong direction.

Some more facts

Namaste means 'I bow to you' and is a greeting for Hindus.

It is like Shalom or 'peace' is for Jews.

It is like Asalaamalaikum or 'peace be upon you' is for Muslims.

It is like Sat Sri Akal or 'God is the ultimate truth' is for Sikhs.

Namaste is spoken with or without a hand gesture made by bringing the palms together at the centre of the chest. I grew up hearing my mum's friends saying it and I've said it back. It's the polite thing to do. It might be two Sanskrit words joined together: *Namah*, meaning 'bow', and *te*, which means 'to you'; together they make for a beautiful and poetic meaning. Some people may disagree, but I would go as far as to say that in India (and when spoken by Hindus elsewhere) Namaste is used in as banal a way as saying hi, hello or good morning (albeit in a highly respectful and formal manner). I suspect this view may divide opinion because I've consulted Hindu friends who agree with me but I've also received messages from people who don't.

My point is that Namaste – pronounced *num us teh*, by the way, not *nama-stay* (I've never heard anyone other than a person with South Asian heritage say it correctly) – has got nothing to do with yoga, and teachers should stop saying it. I've been contacted by white people who say that Indian people in their yoga classes like it when they say it, and I don't doubt that they do. Not all South Asians agree on everything, which might come as a surprise to some people. And there are others who have studied ancient Indian cultures and have argued with me because they claim to have found links between Namaste and yoga. I suspect we won't all ever agree.

Yoga is Egotistic

Or at least some of its teachers and practitioners seem to be. It shouldn't be if we remind ourselves of the Yamas and Niyamas of the Eight Limbs (see page 82). We all have egos, of course, but it seems that many yoga practitioners and teachers devote a lot of time to massaging theirs while channelling gratitude, acceptance and pretending to be on the path to ego-lessness. Yoga teaching should be a service job, in the sense that it's about the people you're tutoring, showing them the ropes and leading the way. Like any other kind of teaching. It's about imparting knowledge – not in the sense that we're better than other people; we might just have a bit more experience with yoga than those we're working with, and our job is to assist them.

This is often referred to as taking yoga off the mat – basically being a good person. Practising yoga postures is a vehicle through which to begin a spiritual journey that involves discipline. But this concept too has become a pastiche of itself since a lot of the people shouting loudest about yoga are those clinging to the image-obsessed version of yoga that we all see everywhere. I'm friends with teachers who aren't like this, and I trained with and have practised with others who've been teaching since the 1980s and 1990s who aren't either.

Teachers with the loudest personalities are also most successful at drawing people to their classes despite not always being the best teachers. The reverse is also true: exceptional teachers can end up teaching very few people. Of course, how popular your class is shouldn't matter. Except it does when you're trying to make a living out of it. Which takes us back to commercialization. Some of the shouty teachers will tell you that yoga isn't just about being flexible (to cover their backs), but they're often the same ones making fancy shapes in photoshoots by poolsides or in front of urban street art.

'I can't tell if they're trying to inspire people to practise yoga or intimidate them,' I said to James, staring at my phone in bed one morning. That's when I first realized that it was me who was intimidated by exactly these people when I started teaching, because if this was what was expected of teachers, there was no way I'd be able to compete.

I once saw a post in a Facebook group, asking for a teacher to lead an online class with a hundred people. There was lots of interest and it got me thinking. When I went to see Beyoncé in concert she didn't know I was there – and this scale of yoga teaching felt a bit like that, except it feels wrong because yoga is not meant to be a performance. When Adriene Mishler, arguably the most famous yoga teacher on YouTube, came to London for an event at Alexandra Palace, there were thousands of people there. At events like this, you're just a body in a sea of bodies. Each to their own, of course, but I don't really understand what the appeal is with this kind of teaching en masse with hundreds of bodies in front of you and at festivals, but that's because being a rock star isn't something I've ever aspired to be. I've been to events like this myself when renowned Ashtanga teacher Richard Freeman was in London in the early noughties, and it was nice to see him and hear from someone who is considered a great master of yoga – but it didn't blow my mind. I turned up, did the thing and left. Freeman was none the wiser. Celebritizing yoga teachers doesn't seem like a good idea. We're not saving lives, though some teachers might swallow the hype (usually their own) and believe they are. Perhaps this trend follows the logical path of social media and the narcissism it can produce in people. Personally, I never film myself practising, but the truth is doing this leads to something more worrying.

Yoga is Sexualized

There are ways in which yoga has become like porn. I've never been into porn. In fact, it puts me off sex more than gets me into it. I'm not even into the feminist stuff. I'm sure that most of us would agree that porn is an idealization of real sex, which can be sloppy, dishevelled, awkward and fumbling. For some it might involve body shame, trigger buried trauma, be over too quickly or not quickly enough. It can be painful, embarrassing, anxiety-inducing and disappointing. It can also be (in my experience, at least) incredibly funny. I had a situation once where a bloke developed a nosebleed (too much cocaine earlier, it turned out), and a giant glob of blood landed on my face, which killed off proceedings. You had to laugh – and I did. But there's nothing funny about the way in which yoga has become sexualized.

Consider how curated our lives are on social media, where you'll find strategically choreographed yoga performed by women wearing bikinis in arse-facing-camera shots. For one thing, these images further serve to distract us from what we're meant to be single-mindedly focused on when practising yoga. That is, liberating ourselves from material things, like bikinis, leggings and the approval of others (this isn't a dig at women, by the way; we should be able to wear and do whatever we want without critique – and it's sad that we often can't). My issue is not so much with what these yogis are wearing. But whether scantily clad or fully clothed, an arse is an arse. Adding an inspirational quote about feeling empowered by your yoga doesn't make it better.

When I posted about this on Instagram, a US-based sex worker with more than a hundred thousand followers shared it to her stories, claiming that 'sensual yoga was still yoga' and that I was policing and perpetuating the idea that 'only skinny people do yoga when everyone can do yoga'. I hope it's clear that she completely missed my point. Others suggested I was wrong because early yogis practised naked thousands of years ago. *So what?* I find myself thinking in response to such comments, because that was then and I'm talking about the present day. In any case, it's not so much the nudity I have a problem with but the posing that comes with it.

I watched one video in which a woman wearing tiny shorts jiggled her bum as she bent over in the bedroom – I was half expecting a bloke hiding behind the door to jump out and 'accidentally' fall on top of her. I showed a friend a couple of accounts on Instagram of yogi women lying on beds, legs splayed or bums facing camera in forward folds (these were allegedly tutorials to help the rest of us civilians practise). 'I'll be honest. I'm a heterosexual man,' he said, 'it's very easy to get turned on, but it also feels uncomfortable. I can't tell if they want me to fancy them or admire their Asanas.'

It's unclear what the people producing this content intend. It does look to me like it's made with an eroticized gaze in mind, and I suspect my friend was uncomfortable because he might have felt things he wasn't expecting to feel (he may have been enjoying those feelings, and perhaps that was the real intention). The point is, the context confused him. Imagine as a straight man putting your yoga kit on and setting your laptop up to start a practice at home. Then being met with that. You'd hardly blame the guy if he couldn't decide whether to reach for his toes or get his cock out. Another friend told me that he tried to be 'a respectful man' in his everyday life, but was worried when he started going to yoga classes that the women would think he was 'some kind of pervert'. 'When I started going to yoga,' he said, 'the first thing some of my friends asked me was whether there were fit women there. They assumed I wasn't there for the yoga.'

Even more ironic is the fact that actual yoga pornography exists. In the name of research I took a look. 'Dirty yoga teacher on fitness model', 'Step-brother massage leads to ripped yoga pants', 'Teen yoga trainer seduces nerd', 'Yoga teacher gets fucked by client', and so on . . . It's all there on Pornhub, and it raises the question whether Pornhub is more honest in its intention than the sexy instructional videos on Instagram. It's not my thing, but you know what you're going to get when you go to a porn site.

The big question, of course, is why some yoga practitioners are presenting themselves this way – in the manner of webcam models. The only answer I've come to is that it's down to an obsession with the body, which comes from the inflated ego and narcissism again. And whether we like it or not – and regardless of the fact that yoga is about liberation (from the bondage of the self, ignorance of the self and material things) – sex will always sell.

Yoga is Voyeuristic

Yoga is sexualized, and this can make the yoga space itself creepy. One day, I was talking to a friend who had been discovering yoga in a big way, which was lovely to hear. She was raving about a teacher (someone I'd seen on Instagram, who was following the trend for photographing and filming students in their classes and then posting the footage online). 'I'm sure he's lovely and reckons he's some kind of spiritual healer or whatever,' I said. 'But he should stop filming his students.'

'What?! I thought he was alright,' she was shocked. I got out my phone and showed her. My friend couldn't believe it.

'It's a weird kind of ownership. Like he's saying: "look at my sleepy children". I don't like it,' she said. When I posted about the issue on social media, I argued that a person's yoga practice is a personal and private matter even when practised in a public place. Teachers don't have the right to document it without permission. If someone took pictures of me in a class without asking, I'd never return. I find it hard to understand why anyone would even want to. The crazy thing was that a couple of teachers who took part in this covert filming 'liked' my post, which is probably a suggestion of their obliviousness. In fact, one of them used to come to that Dharma class I went to. I didn't have the nerve to ask them why they did it.

Yoga is Whatever You Want it to Be

You've possibly heard this on your travels around studios, online tutorials and Instagram. But is it true? It's a convenient notion. The idea being that one could approach any activity yogically: stirring a risotto, washing dishes, hanging out wet clothes to dry. But there's a big difference between doing something with care and attention – mindfully, if you will – and practising yoga.

Mindful walking has become one of my favourite practices to do – but it's still walking. And when it's not yoga, we shouldn't say it is. Yoga people seem to be consistently obsessed with discussing what yoga is. I get the sense that the people most intent on getting to the bottom of it are the ones who also want to reform it. It's the million-rupee question endlessly debated on podcasts and panels, and on social media. Despite this, there's not enough talk about the stuff that matters most. It seems to me that, before it starts becoming something new, yoga needs to remember what it actually is.

Does This Mean It's All Over for Yoga?

I'd like to think not. Yoga has clearly changed, and something of it has died. But the good thing is that many people who work within it are becoming as concerned about it as I am.

A friend who has taught for more than ten years told me that a well-known teacher had told her in confidence that she knew little about the Yoga Sutras and that the academic talk around yoga – the historical and spiritual stuff – goes over her head. This shocked my friend, who felt that studying the texts should be standard practice among teachers. Another senior teacher I know mentioned that a yoga business behind a chain of studios in London had invited teachers to attend meetings on pay but asked them to keep the discussions confidential. The teacher argued that this request was 'an example of ruling by fear and intimidation'. Asteya is the Yama that encourages non-stealing. It's ironic that the behaviour of certain big players profiting from the commerce of yoga might be failing according to that principle and is clearly another area where the yoga industry needs a revamp. It's also a shame that when discussions are raised by people bold enough to do so, they are often shut down or ignored. My yoga teacher friend who wrote to the North London studio named and shamed on Facebook told me she lost a hundred followers after writing a post about white privilege on her social media.

* * *

Not everyone will agree that yoga's riddled with problems, particularly, I suspect, the businesses running wellness empires with money at stake, as well as influencers and trainee teachers who have fled corporate lives for a life spent in the Lotus Pose.

But in some ways the old yoga is over, because what yoga was meant for and intended to be isn't what the practice has now become. Yoga has become disjointed. It's been prised apart and carelessly stuck back together in a new form, which is why we have people misusing language, mistaking the meaning of Namaste, and reimagining Hindu gods as groovy, T-Shirt pin-ups. All of this is why I believe yoga has become a political issue. Some people say that yoga shouldn't be political, but in this day and age – when yoga should be accessible for everyone and anyone but isn't – it can't *not* be political. It's no bad thing if yoga as we currently know it is dead or dying, because it paves the way for a rebirth, and that is definitely something that needs to happen.

CHAPTER 12

Practice and Possibilities

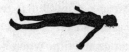

Everybody seems to be terribly interested in yoga. Yoga has become a business affair like everything else. There are teachers of yoga all over the world and they're coining money as usual. Yoga doesn't mean merely to keep your body healthy, normal, active, or intelligent. The meaning of that word in Sanskrit means 'join together'. To have a deeply, orderly, moral, ethical life – not just merely various postures – that was the real meaning of the highest form of yoga.

Jiddu Krishnamurti, philosopher, speaker and writer
(From a public talk in Ojai, California in May 1985[35])

It's fascinating to think that Krishnamurti made this observation about yoga's popularity almost forty years ago. He died the year following that talk in California but clearly saw what was coming for yoga a decade before I discovered the practice myself. I wonder what he would make of what yoga has become today. The yoga industry has become a big beast, so unwieldy that it might seem like there's no way back. But what if we didn't go back and instead looked to a new future?

In my search for what yoga might look like next, I feel hopeful about possibilities for change. When I wrote my piece in *HuffPost* in 2020, I ended it by saying that 'yoga is a political issue and needs a revolution'. It might have sounded radical but I was trying to suggest that a massive shift is needed. Change won't happen overnight, just as it took decades to get from where yoga was at my first class in the nineties to where we are now. But it can and will happen because cultures always evolve.

I discovered Ashtanga at a time when it was hugely popular and was *the* yoga it seemed everyone wanted to do. Over the years it's been outshone by various Vinyasa hybrid styles that are now the classes most in demand. That's not a problem in itself, but add to it the conveyor belt of new training schools that have set themselves up to churn out new yoga teachers accredited by governing bodies that don't always appear to have the most rigorous criteria and have questionable methods for regulating the industry, and it's no surprise that yoga has been watered down so much. Over the years, wellness-focused businesses have also moved in to capitalize on our increased interest in our minds and bodies and appetite for ethical living by selling us the superfoods, cosmetics and apparel we feel we need to be better citizens of the world.

The Big Question: What Now?

The narrative of yoga in the West needs to change in several ways. Firstly, I believe that yoga should be redefined and reformed as the practice for self-inquiry that it was intended as, and not simply be pedalled as a wellness product or method for self-care. Secondly, and perhaps most importantly, yoga must be made available for anyone who wants it in their life. The way it currently stands, it isn't. This is why I feel strongly that yoga will stay a political issue as long as it continues to be commodified, distorted and expensive, and for as long as history, imperialism and colonialism continue to be ignored.

How Can Change Be Achieved?

Returning to what Kehinde Andrews says about the impossibility of trusting anyone who benefits from a structure to change that system, I believe it has to start with each of us on an individual level. We don't have to wait for others who have more influence and power, or to hope for the best – and we shouldn't. Whether we own yoga businesses, are teachers or practitioners, there are things we can all do. Change starts with us. Which brings me to the issue at hand: a manifesto to save yoga from its own success.

Disrupting something as vast as the yoga status quo might sound overwhelming but none of us has to carry the weight of it all on our own shoulders. We don't need massive social media followings or lots of money to get started. It can be as simple as returning to ourselves and thinking about actions we can take in our small corners of the world with the communities we move within. Revolutions happen gradually but they can feel fast once they gather momentum. Small acts add up like tiny grains of sand. The more people involved, the bigger the pile of sand, until it doesn't look anything like what was there before.

Here is my eight-pronged manifesto of how to get started on that change.

The Yoga Manifesto: Eight Pillars (or Limbs) for the Recovery of Yoga

This is less about destroying the old system and more about working together to build a new one. Unlike the Eight Limbs of Yoga, these Pillars aren't designed to be taken in the order that they appear below. This makes them less steps and more areas that I've identified for progress. Ideally, we want all individuals and organizations doing their bit so that slowly they're happening all at the same time. That's when the tide will start to turn. I've listed the Pillars loosely alphabetically so the order they appear in is largely arbitrary. I see them a bit like spokes on a bicycle wheel; they all need to be in place at the same time to hold the wheel in position and keep it moving.

1. Businesses, Brands and Social Media Influencers

I'm not here to put anyone out of business but if change is going to happen, yoga and wellness brands could think about putting their money where their hearts are. By this I mean returning to yogic principles to inspire the way their businesses are run. If they're selling yoga products, they could consider widening their market to include more people. This might mean taking a look at whether what's being sold feels exclusive, expensive or culturally appropriative. Some may already be making efforts to think about how they can do things differently but I wonder if there's more everyone could do. There's no point in hiding behind the fact that yoga is a spiritual practice when ethics get left behind in the way a business makes its money. Activewear and fashion labels should take care with the messaging they use too. There have been many cases of high-profile brands releasing marketing slogans or products that have caused offence, which leaves me wondering how they got out before someone stopped them. This is where hiring a diverse workforce would help and consulting a wide range of voices to ensure no harm is done.

It might sound like a big ask to change business models but it's not impossible. If there's a shift in the intentions of founders, chief executives and managers who have access to large amounts of capital there's no reason why things can't change quickly. Every business will have different needs and abilities to reorganize themselves but one of the most powerful ways they could adapt is to return to yoga philosophy. Applying some of the tenets of yoga – the Yamas and Niyamas – to their business models, specifically Ahimsa (non-violence), Asteya (non-stealing) and Aparigraha (non-greed), would have a big impact on redefining yoga's commercial narrative.

2. Community, Collectives, Union

If we consider what wellness and yoga mean in the broadest sense, I think they imply taking care of ourselves but also looking at how we can keep society well too. This is where collective responsibility becomes important: recognizing that we are part of something and self-reflecting on what we can do to take care of our communities and society as a whole.

This powerful work for change is already in motion in the UK. The Yoga Teachers' Union[36] was established in October 2020 by a collective of teachers to bring about radical change in the yoga community. The union is the first independent body in the UK to recognize that yoga today is no longer a spiritual practice but has become a business. It was set up to campaign so that the industry reflects the principles of liberation at the heart of yoga. They plan to work for fair pay and an end to bullying by employers, which all sounds promising to me.

There's a lot of competitiveness in the yoga industry because it's so big, with businesses vying for the same customers, and teachers going for the same jobs or having to take work they don't enjoy because the pay is so poor. This is where the union comes in. But I also wonder if there are other ways teachers and businesses can collaborate on community initiatives to take yoga to people who can't access or don't feel comfortable in yoga studios. Doing things like making the charity classes I taught better paid, donating mats or other resources to make the practice more enjoyable, or covering costs for nicer venues that aren't crammed with other furniture that has to be pushed to the side, limiting space. This is where if we work with yoga in some way, we can think about small ways we can come together to share the practice with more people, planting seeds and ultimately transforming lives. Yoga means to join together, after all.

3. Diversity, Representation, Equity and Inclusion

This idea is partly an action point and partly something to think about. Accessibility is what I care about most when it comes to yoga, sometimes even more than cultural appropriation, which I've got better at ignoring. This might sound hard to believe given all I've said. It's because I've lost count of the number of people who have told me that for a long time they thought yoga wasn't for people like them (because of alienating images on social media and the way the practice is marketed). I've seen lives change overnight, as mine did after my first yoga class decades ago. This practice is powerful, and more people should be given access to it.

I'd love to see a move away from a one-size-fits-all yoga because it doesn't. It might fit ex-dancers, the hypermobile or those with naturally flexible bodies. But I've never had any of these bodies myself and most people, from what I've seen during my years of teaching classes to the public, don't either. A couple of years ago I was contacted by a young woman who has autonomic dysfunction and fibromyalgia. Both conditions meant that her body was intolerant to some forms of exercise where internal heat would build up, increasing her heart rate, which sometimes caused fainting. She wanted a yoga practice for the physical and mental benefits but told me she felt out of place in yoga classes and thought styles like Ashtanga weren't for people like her. We lived in different parts of the country so we started working together online. I challenged her but without pushing too far, and we had a dialogue that meant that she could regulate what suited her best. I often think of that student when I'm teaching classes in yoga studios and wonder how many others like her don't have the means to access a private teacher or feel out of place in public classes as she did. It might be hard for them to join what's often billed as a mixed-ability, all-levels class, but wouldn't it be great if there was a way to create spaces for people with disabilities or other specific needs? Again, this is something that teachers and community groups could explore with the backing of local businesses to cover wages and pay for resources needed.

When I talk about diversity and representation, I mean it in all forms: gender, sexuality, ethnicity, and all body shapes and sizes. I'm thinking aside from able-bodied people, of those with disabilities, different ages and so on. I've said it before but it's worth saying again that featuring diverse-looking models on marketing (while helpful) isn't quite enough if the yoga being sold isn't serving the people being represented on those flyers and websites. I understand that it's not possible to represent every single person, but having it in mind as a priority changes everything. When you're from a minority, you see lack of diversity everywhere. If you have a business, it would be helpful to look at the workforce, in your classes if you teach, or at the products that you're selling, and think about who you're appealing to. Perhaps notice who is missing. Why aren't they there? Do they even want to be there? Why not? This means brands and businesses should think deeply about what values they're aligned with. They should interrogate who they exist to serve and be honest about whether they're talking to a wide audience or creating invisible barriers that lead to yoga only being available to some parts of society and being taken away from others. Investing in projects that help take yoga to low-income and hard-to-reach communities, and paying teachers fairly so they can do this, is one way to help change this. Yoga teachers, too – look at your classes. Is the language you use welcoming and inclusive? Is there equality and fairness in the room? Are you taking care of everyone?

4. History and Imperialism, Colonialism, and Cultural Appropriation

There isn't much more for me to say about these concepts other than to state how important it is to be aware of them all. The history of yoga, what it is and where it comes from, is important to understand, as is modern South Asia and its bloody history due to being colonized. Many of the strange and uncomfortable experiences I had as a yoga teacher were down to me being a South Asian woman working in a white yoga world. At times I felt it was a bit like 'selling yoga back to South Asians' by people who thought they knew more about it. In some cases that may have been true; there are many white teachers who will have studied more deeply than me. But there's a strange power dynamic at play that I can never put my finger on. I think it probably has to do with me being a descendent of a land and people that was colonized. This isn't anyone else's fault, but it's a fact that could be handled with greater awareness and sensitivity. This goes back to thinking about yoga not just as a wonderful ancient practice but looking at it within the context of the world we live in.

My advice to teachers, practitioners and businesses with yoga-related Sanskrit names is to be cautious, humble, sensitive and welcoming. Acknowledge the culture you're promoting, rather than burying the connection or pretending it was yours all along. At the same time, I find it unhelpful when I see gatekeeping of yoga by other groups. This could be a backlash against the global commodification and whitewashing of yoga but I still don't agree with it. My main message here, as before, is anyone can practise yoga if they want to – of course you don't have to be South Asian – but I think it's important we all do it with integrity and respect.

I think cultural appropriation will always be a tricky area for many of us. It's not always easy to work out whether we're on the right side of it, but there are examples that are blindingly obvious, as I explained earlier. I think a key thing to remember with all of this is that you don't have to pretend you're not culturally appropriating, or get defensive if you're called out. Being aware that it's easy to do, and committing to trying to avoid it at all costs, is already heading in the right direction.

I've seen calls to decolonize yoga, which is a sentiment I understand, but that word has never really chimed with me. I'm not entirely sure that's possible anyway because India has been invaded thousands of time in history. I'd rather focus on a brand new revolutionized yoga rather than one that's defined by its past colonization.

5. Outreach

I've already referred to this in terms of individuals and organizations coming together to work within communities, but here's an example of a successful one that I know more about. My friend Amani who taught me about Egyptian Yoga in Chapter 4 (see page 96) founded a charity called Project Yogi, running classes for children and young people in schools across London. She came across similar problems to those that I did when I was teaching those refugee classes. I asked what led to her moving into this work.

I think yoga spaces are still very white and I know that some of the people running these places want to be more diverse and attract people of colour into their spaces, but it is going to take time and more than their staff taking diversity training, although that is a start. Some studios don't have enough Black teachers or teachers of colour. I think they need to switch it up and have a variety. Yoga spaces will be more welcoming to students of colour if they do that. That said, taking a few pictures of Black people doesn't change things. I'm hopeful the image of yoga will change but it will take time.

I asked her what she thinks it will take for things to change.

Proper change needs to involve outreach. If I take it back to Project Yogi – the whole idea was to always work with under-represented and underprivileged groups. But a big problem we faced at the start was that they were not always interested in coming. You can't just make something low-cost or free and expect people to come, and money is not always the issue. There has to be outreach, to pull them in. This is why with Project Yogi we go into schools to speak directly to communities we can support. The solution for making yoga more accessible is outreach, genuine care and community cohesion.

Yoga's popularity has brought with it the issue of it being taken away from some communities who might get some value from it, but Amani's doing something about it.

6. Students

As students, you should feel free to question everything. After my classes I always invite people to come and ask me anything, and I never mind if I don't know the answer. If it's a question about a posture we can work it out together or if it's a philosophical point I'll think about it or look it up. That's how I keep learning.

I know firsthand that many students want more from yoga because they've often come to me saying they want to practise yoga in a more conscientious way. Many have told me they want to get to the heart of what the practice is, away from the fancy activewear and homogenized clichés that the practice is only suitable for bendy, acrobatic, able-bodied people. It doesn't have to be like this. It's really important that it doesn't stay like this – for everyone, but especially for young people like the teenage boys I met at the beginning of this book. This also makes me think about teenage me and how unwell I was when my mum took me to my first class. If she took me to a mainstream class now, I wonder whether I would go back. The sad fact is that if I started my yoga journey now I think I would struggle to find my place and would probably feel intimidated and confused about what yoga is and how it might help me. It would mean missing out on finding the powerful tools this practice can offer.

As I said before, my take on yoga isn't the only way and won't work for everyone, but my key message here is that as students we don't have to blindly follow teachers, who are on their own paths as well. They're flawed; we all are. Teachers are there to guide and show us the way, but ultimately this practice is about thinking for ourselves. If we return to the Eight Limbs and think about Svadhyaya (self-study) and also Tapas (austerity/overcoming adversity/transformation), this is work that we must do independently.

In the same way that we might support sustainable fashion or think about where we buy our groceries and be conscious of purchasing single-use plastic, as practitioners we can also think about which businesses we are prepared to uphold through where we choose to practise yoga. As students we can also do our research, and ask our teachers about their own practice and training so we know who we're learning from. I'm always happy to speak about my background if anyone asks because I've undergone several training courses and gained certificates but I've also lived a life with yoga, and it gives me an opportunity to talk about that too, which feels important when it comes to teaching.

7. Studios

I tend to avoid most yoga studios these days unless I'm there to practise with a teacher I like, or I'm there to teach, and if I'm doing that it's likely to be somewhere that I like the ethos of. I love the classes I currently teach and now only teach in places where I feel at home and have the autonomy to teach how I want to. But I'd say yoga studios are generally not places that I belong. There are plenty of things studios can do to improve. Many already offer community classes that cost less but are often held during the day on weekdays, which makes me wonder how helpful they are for people who need to work. When I was growing up, my single mum wouldn't have been able to go to a daytime community class. She wouldn't have been able to go in the evenings either when I was home from school, but I'm sure there will be others for whom out-of-office times do work. This requires studios to tap into their surrounding communities to discover the needs of people who live nearby and how to serve them better so those people are coming through the doors. I know there is an interest in yoga that's wider than the people going to yoga studios because of all the community groups I've taught and what I saw through working in leisure centres.

Offering subsidised spots during peak times could be something worth trying, as would prioritizing teaching opportunities for teachers of colour – South Asian ones in particular. This links back to the diversity issue outlined above in point 3. Yoga teachers also deserve fairer pay. Norman told me about several London studios he had gathered information on where the pay structures had not been changed for at least ten years.[37] This was despite classes costing more. When business booms and class prices are hiked up, teachers' pay could also be improved. Since the COVID pandemic in 2020, with some studios forced to close, classes slashed or poorly attended, and pay reduced when it wasn't great in the first place, things have got worse for teachers working for big businesses.[38] It might sound reasonable for wages to be cut when businesses have seen a decline in profits. I don't think it is. When you teach yoga you're paid only for the length of the class, not the time it takes to get to the venue, set up or chat to students afterwards. That's a lot of time and teachers do it because they love to. They should be remunerated better. It's the right thing to do in accordance with the ethics of yoga.

8. Teachers and Teacher Training

As yoga teachers we can think about the wider yoga system we are part of, who we're working for, how and what we're teaching. We can offer ideas to the studios we work at, and raise some of the issues such as diversity and inclusion, or history and cultural appropriation. We can take more interest in the bigger picture rather than just thinking about our own classes. I realize that rocking the boat with employers isn't easy; I didn't speak up straight away as I was too busy trying to make ends meet. Then when I did take action (over the incident with Rachel, see page 142), it didn't work. That's what led to writing this book. It's my contribution to kick-start the revolution. I knew I wasn't going to be a career teacher after I left my job at the yoga studio. I never wanted that anyway, but I was tired of imposter syndrome, and my desire to tell the truth outdid my need to fit in. Speaking out as I did on social media carved out my own path. The more I did it I realized it was the only way forward. Being honest was a risk but it has also opened up opportunities. It's led to collaborations with others on community-based projects that feel close to my heart, it's seen me being offered classes to teach *because* of my political stance on yoga and not despite it. I've led workshops with teachers on some of the problematic issues such as the commercialization of yoga, cultural appropriation and inclusion that I've discussed in this book, and I have been invited to speak at events. These are ways that I've been finding my feet away from the mainstream yoga scene that I didn't feel part of for so long and now have no desire to be. There are ways we can all find our path as teachers and work in ways that feel right to us or might be better for living according to the practice.

Speaking of teaching, yoga teacher training providers could consider revising their course syllabuses to include modules that cover some of the issues I discussed in chapter 11. I saw this work well when I was invited to be one of the lead facilitators of a four-month teacher training that started in January 2022 in London. As well as teaching the mandatory theory and postural practice to be expected on such courses, I led discussions on yoga philosophy that took a close look at how the ancient wisdom might apply to modern life. These discussions led to questions and conversations among the students around diversity and inclusion, colonialism, cultural appropriation and more. The sessions were energizing, rich with ideas and felt important for the future of yoga teaching and what happens to the practice next. Other training providers could do the same.

The US-based Yoga Alliance is the world's largest accreditor of yoga training and has strict criteria for courses. Yoga studios will usually only hire you if you've undergone a training that has been approved by them. All but one of the training courses I have done were YA certified, which means that the number of hours I have trained aren't all accounted for under this system. This doesn't matter to me personally, but it's important if you're a new teacher. It also became important when I was hired to work on the teacher training that I helped facilitate (January–April 2022) and had to prove that I had taught a certain number of hours in order to qualify for an Experienced Yoga Teacher badge. Without that I wouldn't have been able to take the job.

I wonder whether there could be a more qualitative approach to assessing training courses that doesn't reduce them to the number of hours trained. Perhaps a person's own experience of yoga outside of official courses could count towards qualifications, which might open yoga teaching work to people who can't afford to pay for expensive courses or indeed YA membership. I also think thirty-day crash courses are to be avoided at all costs and should be abolished, but perhaps that's wishful thinking.

* * *

These eight pillars might seem like a mountain to climb. They're just ideas and they might not all work. There may be resistance and it might take time for people to become willing, but I hope they provide something to think about. Thinking about change is also a step in the right direction. Then starting to take action somewhere – anywhere, in however small a way – will build momentum and reveal other creative ways to change things for good.

It was necessary for me to unpack all of this to make sense of the practice and what it means to me and to process the confusions of the yoga industry that I discovered by working as a teacher. It's because I feel so deeply for this practice that I have spent so much time in this book trying to speak honestly about how things could be better.

It might seem like too great a feat to burst the yoga bubble but in a way it already has burst. I'm not the only person who wants to see a change within yoga. There are many others who teach and practise yoga across the world who are actively starting to use their voices and platforms to open conversations, create opportunities and push for change in their communities. That's how revolutions start, and they progress when we work together. There is a fresh zeitgeist emerging as new voices come forward and more community-focused independent yoga teachers realize their own power and make their voices heard. The more of us who choose to get involved in this work, the greater our influence, and soon those with more power such as big businesses might join the movement.

Not long ago I was invited to speak on a panel to discuss what it means to take care of ourselves. The idea was to look at what it means to thrive, within the context of social media's favourite wellness hashtag – #selfcare. The Chair opened the conversation by asking all panellists what self-care meant to us. It struck me that being asked to speak about self-care as someone who for a very long time didn't know how to do it felt like a strange thing. I'm still working it out and wasn't immediately sure what I might say. At the same time, you might have arrived at the end of this book with a sense that I'm someone who is anti-wellness, and in a sense you would be right – I am. It's because yoga and wellness seem to be oppressive industries that are rigged in their exclusive design to serve only the privileged. I could have talked about yoga and everything it's done for me personally but I wouldn't have been able to do that without talking about the times it hasn't worked. I started to wonder if I even knew what self-care was. I knew it wasn't to do with scented candles, spa days, expensive activewear and pricey yoga memberships (as great as these things might be).

Luckily, I was sitting at the end of the row of speakers on the stage so I had a moment to gather my thoughts. I reflected on how self-care has changed so much throughout life. It didn't exist in my younger years when I wasn't eating properly, and that form of self-harm dragged itself into my thirties when I was drinking heavily. I have had different needs at various points of my life. The same might be true for you. What we need when we're physically or mentally unwell will differ from when we're stressed, going through a relationship break-up, are bereaved, or have had an exhausting day.

As I picked up my mic to speak on the panel, I realized that what I've needed for my own self-care when I've been in a bad spot in life has been other people. I've had to be social and to engage in the world to balance out my tendency to isolate, but I also have to know when to withdraw to stop myself going into overwhelm. The same goes for my practice. Yoga is a deeply personal practice for me, as you know. But as personal as it is, I wouldn't have got very far with my practice without community and somewhere to belong. Teaching yoga has been about relationships too. Neither teaching yoga nor practising it has ever been about escaping society. They've both been about learning how to live with myself so that I can be a better part of it. In this way, while I don't think self-care is selfish, I believe it has to extend into looking after ourselves to take care of the world around us, too.

It took a long time for me to understand that this was what the practice was for. I've learnt lessons from gifted yoga teachers and fellow students on their own paths, which has taught me about the strength to be found in being part of a collective. That progress is possible when we're together and not pushing against adversity and hardships alone, which I have spent a long time trying to do. Thích Nhất Hạnh says it well: 'It is difficult if not impossible to practise the way of understanding and love without a sangha, a community of friends who practise the same way'.[39] In other words, we need each other to succeed.

There's a saying in the recovery fellowships that I attended years ago that 'you can't bullshit a bullshitter', the idea being that we've all lied to others and ourselves when we were deep in the throes of self-destruction, so there's no point in lying to each other. The only way to recover is to speak our truth.

So what self-care boils down to for me is honesty. Having close friends who I can be honest with and a great therapist to help me make sense of life. Both of these things are crucial because when I can be honest with others, I'm honest with myself. This is important because many years went by where I was shrouded in guilt and shame and couldn't be honest at all. So for me, self-care starts with telling the truth.

My desire to speak the truth in this book has been a form of self-care too. This practice that I befriended very early in life, then stuck with, discarded and returned to more times than I can count, has carried me through life but my relationship with it has changed many times. This is why giving you an honest take on yoga as well as showing how I've seen the practice evolve and suggesting ways I believe it needs to transform yet again felt so important.

It's a fertile time for change. A hashtag might not change the world, despite my flippant claim years ago, but people can and always do. Yoga is a practice for learning about and transforming ourselves, after all. We can also use it to transform the world. The only solution is revolution and change is down to us. There will be peaks and troughs and moments of serendipity along the way. Get involved in whatever way feels right. Make loads of mistakes and then make some more. Learn, grow, move forward.

Over to you.

In the Beginning Was the Word, and the Word Was Om

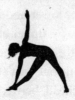

This is a by no means exhaustive, short introduction to common yoga-related words that are useful to know.

Ashtanga: *Ash* means 'eight', *tanga* means 'limbs'. It commonly refers to the dynamic set of postures that I've mentioned throughout this book, but in terms of Patanjali's Yoga Sutras, it refers to the principles laid out to internally purify the body and mind in order to reveal the universal self and find enlightenment.

Aum/Om: This is said to be the origin of all sounds and the seed of creation.

Asana: This translates as 'seat', but the more modern interpretation of the word denotes physical postures or poses.

Bandha: These are internal muscular 'locks' that, when engaged, support the toning and lifting of strategic areas of the body. The three major bandhas are: Mula Bandha – the pelvic floor muscles; Uddiyana Bandha – the abdominals up to the diaphragm; and Jalandhara Bandha – the throat.

Chakra: The word means 'wheel' and these are energy centres in the body located between the base of the spine and the top of the head. We are believed to have seven and each is associated with a different colour:

root (Muladhara) – base of the spine (red)
sacral (Svadhisthana) – lower abdomen (orange)
solar plexus (Manipura) – upper abdomen (yellow)
heart (Anahata) – centre of the chest (green)
throat (Vishuddha) – throat area (blue)
Third Eye (Ajna) – forehead, between the eyebrows (purple)
crown (Sahasrara) – the very top of the head (violet, also sometimes white).

Drishti: Refers to a focal point or gaze point when doing yoga poses. The reason we send the gaze to the belly button, big toe or space between the feet is to narrow the focus of the mind. Sending the gaze to the navel is the tradition but unlikely to work for everyone. In Downward Facing Dog these days I tend to look at the space between my feet. It feels more natural and I often suggest this to students I teach. Otherwise I encourage them to rest their gaze wherever it is comfortable, because it doesn't matter. The main thing is for the gaze to be still because if the eyes are moving the mind is likely to follow. During meditation, we frequently send the 'internal gaze' to the space between the forehead where the Third Eye (seat of intuition) is said to rest.

Chaturanga Dandasana: Four-limbed/legged Stick Pose or low plank. There are a lot of Chaturangas in Ashtanga and Vinyasa classes!

Downward Facing Dog (Adho Mukha Svanasana): This is one of the most common yoga poses, and looks like an upside-down 'V' shape.

Eight limbs: The steps to enlightenment: Yama, Niyama, Asana, Pranayama, Pratyahara, Dharana, Dhyana, Samadhi.

Hatha: In Sanskrit, *Ha* represents 'sun' and *tha* represents 'moon'. Hatha forms the basis for most styles of yoga, and is often used to describe slower-paced classes with no flow to them. Hatha is pronounced *Hata*. The 't' is aspirated which makes the 'h' silent, as in the word 'Thai' as opposed to 'think'.

Kundalini: This refers to spiritual energy that is believed to have been coiled at the base of the spine since birth, and is the source of the life force or prana (see below), also called Chi in Chinese traditions.

Lokah Samastah Sukhino Bhavantu: This is the last line of the Ashtanga closing chant and loosely translated as: 'May all beings everywhere be happy and free'. It's a very common chant in its own right with a lovely sentiment that is sometimes emblazoned on sweatshirts. I sold one for £70 when I worked at my yoga studio job. Quite ironic, given this phrase's popularity, that there is such inequality and disparity within the yoga industry itself.

Mudra: This is a hand gesture used to aid concentration and facilitate the flow of energy or prana (see below) in the body.

Namaste: Okay, so you know we don't need this one anymore. But see more on page 259 if you want to know why.

Prana: This is life energy, life force within the body.

Patanjali: He was the sage from the third or second century BCE said to have compiled the Yoga Sutras, which are philosophical texts containing a guide on how to live and advance along a spiritual path towards enlightenment. It's not known if Patanjali was one person or many.

Pranayama: These are breathing exercises that clear the physical and emotional obstacles in our body to free the breath and flow of prana.

Satya: Truth – telling it, living it, owning it.

Savasana: This means Corpse Pose or Dead Body Pose, typically at the end of a yoga class, though in India it was common with some teachers I practised with to both start and end the class with this posture. I often think of this posture as being the ideal place for Samadhi (see Eight Limbs above) should it come. For me Savasana represents the unifying aspects of yoga, so in a sense there's no body, and no mind. There's nothing left of me but the breath or prana.

Seva: This usually means service, or I sometimes interpret it as participation, being useful, helping out. Service has a big emphasis in recovery fellowships, where everyone is there to help one another. Others take on commitments to help run the meetings. Yoga teaching too can be seen as a service job, particularly if you're volunteering. But it could also mean being a supportive friend, neighbour, member of your community.

Shaanti: Peace, so the common chant *Om, shaanti, shaanti, shaanti*, means 'Om, peace, peace, peace'.

Surya Namaskar (Sun Salutation): This is a dynamic sequence of postures often used to warm up the body at the start of a yoga class. In Ashtanga there are two versions, A and B. When I'm travelling or feeling jetlagged, I will often just practise five of each and then do the Ashtanga finishing sequence so that I still maintain my practice even when I have less time. I recommend this for beginners and indeed whenever I meet someone who is injured, low on energy or having a rough emotional time. Less can be plenty.

Ujjayi: This can be commonly translated as the 'victorious breath' or 'oceanic breath' because of the sound the breath makes on the exhale through a slightly constricted throat.

Vinyasa: In Sanskrit this roughly translates as 'to move in a special way' and typically describes movement between held poses. When describing a yoga class, it refers to a style where movement is linked with the breath, as it is in Ashtanga but the poses will be in a different order. In Vinyasa classes, postures are strung together in a short or longer flow.

Yang yoga: This is often used to describe a style of yoga that is more rhythmic, repetitive and energetic – great for building strength and flexibility and for focus. It could apply to any number of yoga styles in the world today (see page 291 for more about them).

Yin yoga: This floor-based meditative practice incorporates principles of Traditional Chinese Medicine while targeting the fascia and connective tissues in the body.

Yoga: The word itself means to 'yoke' or 'bind' – often interpreted as 'union' (the union of body and mind).

Twenty-three Styles of Yoga

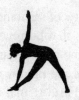

I've lost count of the number of people who have come to me filled with questions about the difference between classes they see on studio timetables. There are many forms of yoga and none of them is better than any other, although some stay closer to the roots of the practice than others.

The best practice is the one that works for you. I may be dismissive of some of the styles we have today but that's not to put you off; I'm just keen for you to better understand what you're practising. So let's go through some of them.

1. Ashtanga Vinyasa
A powerful and dynamic style that follows a systematic set sequence. Most drop-in classes will follow the Primary Series, though there's never time to do it all in a standard hour or 75 minute class. There are six series in total and I suspect very few living people have mastered them all. It's physically challenging but, as the sequence and postures become familiar, it can become deeply meditative. You won't find any music. You're encouraged to use the *Ujjayi* (victorious) *Pranayama* (breathing technique) as you move, which creates a shallow

oceanic wave-like sound. The breath becomes the soundtrack. It's imperative to mention that the man who popularized this method, Pattabhi Jois, turned out to be a sexual abuser (see page 145). This was revealed in 2018, creating divisions among Ashtangis and throwing the global community of practitioners into crisis.

The perceived rigidity of Ashtanga is what has led to offshoots of other styles that borrow from this one but take on different names. Some of them are below. It's also interesting to me that it was the rigidity rather than the scandal around Jois that emerged in 2018 that seems to be the principal cause of Ashtanga falling out of fashion.

2. (Mysore-style) Ashtanga Self-practice

The first thing that washes over you when you step into a Mysore room is the silence – apart from the sound of *Ujjayi* breathing. Even though everyone is moving, there is a stillness in the air. It's called Mysore-style after its place of origin in India. It's Ashtanga but with a difference. You practise the sequence outlined above but at your own pace within a group setting. The teacher usually opens the class with a chant and then moves around the room like a silent angel, offering one-to-one tuition and hands-on adjustments. The teacher then adds new postures from the Ashtanga system to the sequence that you're practising as you progress. This method of practising alone in a group environment allows you to tune into your own body and experience more profoundly. Assisting can be a deeply powerful exchange in the Mysore room – it's a dialogue. It's also about trust. It's important to know that you can refuse adjustments too, and when I assist I always ask if students want them. Mysore-style is traditionally practised in the early morning so it's not for everyone.

3. Bikram and Hot Yoga

Another style that isn't for everyone. Bikram is usually done in a room heated to 36–40°C so you spend a lot of time dribbling into your mat. Aside from the fact that the man who created this is an alleged sexual abuser too (see page 150), the sequence never made sense to me because you go from standing to lying down to standing up again, which seems like a waste of energy. Plus you do every single pose twice, so don't go if you get bored easily. I went through a hot yoga phase late in my yoga journey when I stopped drinking in June 2016. It wasn't Bikram but a franchise company that offered a slightly more interesting sequence and range of poses. The heat helped calm my nerves because I was perpetually anxious and had the shakes. It did the trick. But Bikram Yoga is purely exercise, in my view, and I generally think that yoga and saunas are probably best done separately. Many hot yoga teachers in my experience also sound like they've memorized a handbook of instructions for directing people into poses. You won't get any adjustments here either – I suppose it's because we're sweating so much and teachers don't want to get involved in that. But I found this lack of personal touch dull. You need a lot of equipment for hot yoga, unless you want to pay for a mat and towel rental and buy two litres of water in a plastic bottle at the studio at every visit. I took my own, which means a lot of lugging stuff around. No pain, no gain.

4. Budokon

This is a yoga and martial arts mash-up that's fitness-based. I've watched videos of people doing it online and *Cor, I wish I could do that* is what comes to my mind. It looks incredible. Founded by a guy called Cameron Shayne, it's loved by Hollywood A-listers including Jennifer Aniston, Courtney Cox, and Rene Russo. I'd hazard a guess that this is because of what Budokon does for their bodies. It's said that a typical session begins with yoga Sun Salutations to lighten and open the body, followed by a martial arts segment of primal dance-like movement (this is what gave me the wow factor). The classes end with a guided meditation. It looks beautiful, like the Brazilian martial art Capoeira. There is a fluidity to it. However, I'm just not sure I understand where it fits in with yoga philosophy.

5. Buti Yoga

Buti is a Marathi Indian term that can be translated as meaning 'the cure to something that's been hidden away or secret'. I've never tried this one but it's a fitness-style method that combines yoga postures with tribal-inspired dancing, plyometric exercises and intentional shaking intended to spark off healing on an emotional and energetic level. It was founded by celebrity trainer Bizzie Gold in 2012, who said in a 2018 blog on her website butiyoga.com that 'tribal does not simply refer to Native American and African tribes'. She goes on to say: 'It is unfair and ignorant to state that the word tribal is somehow wrong, politically incorrect or offensive. Tribal dance in our case may refer to aspects of Hawaiian, Tahitian, West African, East African . . . we've even seen Ukrainian traditional dance and other Eastern European cultural dances. I'm a Hungarian Jew and we refer to ourselves as a tribe and have traditional dances.'[40] It sounds fun but I'm not sure it's still yoga with so much else going on. Who knows? I'll let you decide.

6. Creative Flow (also Mindful Flow, Aroma Flow)

I asked a teacher who taught Creative Flow to tell me more. She said: 'It looks like yoga but it isn't.' It's a freestyle movement class, from what I've since seen. It tends to be less about holding poses and more about exploring the spaces between them, which brings to mind the concept of negative space in art. Negative space is the space around an object, not the thing itself. This is a fascinating thing to explore from a creative and embodiment of body point of view. It shifts your perspective, and I can see how this style could be a deeply soulful experience for some. It's empowering to move freely and explore your body, how it feels and what it might do, without having to form poses. Creative Flow feels removed from the notion of discipline, which I'm drawn to, and I think I'd probably be happier dancing 5Rhythms,[41] a transformative movement meditation practice that I love devised by Gabrielle Roth in the late 1970s. Aroma classes add on a layer of essential oils, and Mindful Flows are just slower (although the teacher might also blend in some other practices like Qi Gong if they want to).

7. Dharma

Developed by Dharma Mittra, a Brazilian based in New York City. The practice is not for the faint-hearted – there is a big emphasis on back bending and a lot of advanced headstands. In my experience, you rarely sit on the floor and there is little in the way of forward bending. Though the class is led in the usual way, there are pauses for you to practise at your own pace while the teacher comes around to assist. It's physically demanding and you would have to be fairly able-bodied and not suffer from any illnesses that affect your energy levels because it demands a lot of effort to move in this way. I got into Dharma in a big way for a while – the back bending supports where I am at in my Ashtanga practice. There's also a strong spiritual focus on cultivating compassion within yourself and spreading it through the world.

8. Flow/Vinyasa Flow

From what I can tell, Flow is stuck on the end of class names to help them sell, as in: Dynamic Flow, Hatha Flow, Vinyasa Flow. In simple terms it's like Ashtanga with the furniture (poses) moved around. I went to a lot of Vinyasa-style classes in my first ten years of practising yoga before I settled on Ashtanga. It's the most popular style of class in the West, or in classes run by Westerners in Eastern countries that I've visited. There's a lot of choreography and the sequence can be whatever the teacher wants it to be. In my experience, you don't stay in each individual pose long enough to get any significant benefit. Flow also conjures up a 1960s long-haired, free-love, hippie image for me, which seems to be what the people (mostly women) going to these classes want. I used to want to be this woman too for a long time but gave up when I realized I'd never make it.

9. Hatha

Probably the most classic form of yoga, from which everything follows. This is where it all started for me with yoga at the YMCA in the 1990s. The poses in all the styles listed here are Hatha yoga in that sense: a Tree Pose is Hatha, as are Triangle and Warrior Poses. There are many more that are too. Those early classes set me up for the rest of my life because I became familiar with lots of the traditional poses without any of the modern distractions of music or complex choreography.

10. Iyengar

Internationally respected for its rigorous approach. It was founded by B.K.S. Iyengar, one of the most influential yoga teachers in the world. It's heavily alignment-obsessed and focused on precision. This will appeal to a lot of people because you can check in with your own body and do what's appropriate (though we should be doing this in other methods of practice too). I know lots of teachers who love it and there is a huge physical benefit to working in this way. I never got into it because I like my regular practice to keep moving rather than getting bogged down in alignment detail. I'm fascinated by anatomy, and have enjoyed Iyengar in a workshop setting, but my principle aim when on the mat is to do the poses and meditation with minimal interruption.

11. Jivamukti
If you're familiar with Ashtanga you'll recognize this. It was started by a New York couple, Sharon Gannon and David Life, who are also vegan campaigners. I went to their original yoga centre in Union Square in New York in 2013 every day for a week and had a good time. There are no mirrors in the changing rooms, which I figure has some spiritual reasoning behind it. There were also 'guru cards' featuring pictures of both Gannon and Life, available in the gift shop, which I found weird. *Jiva* is a bhakti devotional practice. Most teachers of this style are into chanting and offer it in their classes. There's a strong sense of community among them, though ego emerges too. It's very physical, which I responded to, but I was drinking heavily in my Jiva years so was probably hungover in most classes I went to. There's always music, and the teacher I went to had some excellent playlists and it sometimes felt like we were clubbing.

12. Smai Tawi, Kemetic or Egyptian Yoga
An ancient Egyptian practice that offers physical postures, breathwork and meditation as well as philosophy and guidance for how to live one's life. One of the modern versions

of Smai Tawi was developed through research conducted by Dr Asar Hapi and Master Yirser Ra Hotep (Elvrid Lawrence) of Chicago in the 1970s. I went to a couple of classes with a lovely teacher on a retreat a few years ago. It was interesting to approach yoga in a new way; some poses were new to me and others were familiar but had different names. There are also lots of hand gestures, which in the Indian system are called mudras. I enjoyed visiting it as another way to explore a spiritual practice that has parallels with South Asian yoga.

13. Kundalini

From what I can see, this is popular among recovering addicts. The breathwork alone can take you to altered states so it appeals to me (in theory at least). The first class I attended with a friend in 2008 was too intense and I never went back because the Pranayama (breathwork) practices were too over-whelming.

It was developed by Yogi Bhajan who brought the practice to the West in 1969. It features Pranayama, mudras, Asana, and meditation. A lot of the teachers wear turbans and many adopt Sikh names. I'm intrigued by this method because it feels like transformation is likely to be strong here. I hope I'm at a place to try this practice again at some point.

14. Mandala

A Mandala is a geometric configuration of symbols used in the Indian religions of Hinduism, Buddhism and Jainism. It can be seen as a model for organizational structure of the Self and the universe. The graphic symbol is usually in the form of a circle divided into four separate sections. In turn, Mandala classes are based on one of the four elements – earth, air, fire or water – and the sequence of poses involves flowing through them and moving in a circle around your mat. I went to a class at the studio where I worked, and found the choreography too fussy – moving around the mat in a 360° circle confused me.

The origins of Mandala yoga are unclear. A lot of teachers working in London who teach it appear to have gone to the same training school, and this school's website put me off with its pictures of the semi-nude founder wearing what appears to be latex or a bondage outfit. I also saw details about shamanic courses and cacao ceremonies, and people wearing Native American headpieces with tribal markings on their faces. I closed the tab on my laptop.

15. Power Yoga

This is another reworked version of Ashtanga, which aims to build flexibility and strength. It looks to me like it's very much focused on the physical as opposed to the spiritual. That said, the Power Yoga Company in London describes itself as: 'Weaving ancient yogic philosophy into 21st century life.'[42] Meanwhile, fitness-studio chain Frame describes its Power Yoga[43] classes as: 'a strong and sweaty class. Expect to challenge yourself throughout, both mentally and physically with long holds, strong balances and advanced options'. So to me it sounds like Ashtanga or Vinyasa Flow but rearranged and with a new name. It's a class that's marketed to gymgoers and high-intensity exercise lovers – essentially people who like to feel like they're working out. I like working strongly and sweating from practising poses too, but I'd rather go to a circuit-training class if exercise is all that we're going to be doing.

16. Restorative

The ultimate in #selfcare. A floppy relaxing class with loads of props and lying around on bolsters. It's an antidote for those of us who live in cities and are perpetually stressed and need somewhere to go where we can pay to take a rest. I took my mum to a three-hour workshop one Mother's Day to force her to lie down. She needed it and loved it. I got bored, but I see the value in this practice. During the 2020 pandemic, when I and many other yoga teachers held live yoga classes online, I sometimes turned what was meant to be a Yin class (see below) into Restorative if that's what I could see people needed. It's actually a huge honour to be with people while they rest, to watch them sink deeper and trust you to stay with them. It's a brilliant way to calm the nervous system and focus on your breath, if your brain isn't shouting at you as is often the case for me. That said, you can practise watching your thoughts, which is a useful exercise too. Or you can take a nap. I prefer Yoga Nidra (see below).

17. Rocket

Inaugurated by Larry Schultz, a California known as 'the bad boy of yoga' because he had a penchant for a spliff and a desire to play around with the Ashtanga series. Larry trained with Pattabhi Jois, the big daddy of Ashtanga mentioned above, and built the Rocket from there. Inspired by Ashtanga but remixed, Rocket Yoga focuses on a sequence of standing, seated and inverted postures and loads of arm-balances and back bends from the more advanced Ashtanga series. It's called the Rocket because it 'gets you there *faster*'. But where is everyone trying to get to? I asked a Rocket teacher once. Turns out that 'there' is a handstand. As with most classes, quality of class does depend on the teacher. I can see its appeal for people bored of Ashtanga or who have unfulfilled ambitions to be gymnasts. I went to a workshop with a wonderful Rocket teacher who taught from the heart and I enjoyed his playful but dignified approach, then I went to another very acrobatty look-what-I-can-do class with a narcissist and never went back.

18. Scaravelli

Inspired by the teachings of Vanda Scaravelli, an Italian yoga teacher who pioneered the idea of effortless yoga. I've been to one class, and I found it gentle on the body, developing core strength, releasing tension and creating length in the spine. This is what I'd regard as the focus of most classes, and Scaravelli is just another way of doing it. The teacher's outlook was that 'there is no age to yoga. You can start at seventy, eighty because if it's done with gravity and breath you receive and you don't go against, you will never damage the body', and this view is to be commended in terms of making yoga accessible.

19. Sivanada

A classical and holistic approach to Hatha Yoga founded by Swami Vishnudevananda in India. His noble aim was to spread the teachings of yoga and the message of world peace. I did lots of it in South India while travelling there because Ashtanga was hard to find. Some of the sequencing felt strange – there's a headstand in the middle, for example (in Ashtanga this comes at the end). Strange doesn't mean wrong, just different. Sivanada's reach is wide so it's popular with a lot of people. I didn't take to it, but I applaud its authenticity and that it draws from yoga philosophy.

20. Yin

My mum took me to my first Yin class in December 2012 when I was double hungover from two days of Christmas lunches. I hated it at first because I felt ill but now, years later, I love it. It's a great antidote to dynamic Asana practices. It's not Indian in its lineage: it draws from Daoism, which is Chinese. Yin was founded by Paulie Zink, a US martial arts champion. The postures are floor-based and aimed at getting into the connective tissue – fascia – that surrounds muscles. It's calming and meditative and, although it is named Yin Yoga, I've often questioned whether it should be called yoga at all. I refer to it as simply Yin to keep it distinct from the South Asian practices when I'm talking about or teaching it. It's also distinct from Restorative Yoga because here there is a focus on holding postures and going to an edge where you experience sensation – and that can sometimes be uncomfortable. Restorative Yoga's aim is to be as comfortable as possible.

21. Yogasana

A Vinyasa hybrid. This is a strong practice that involves moving in a choreographed way from one pose to the next. The class is usually sweaty. It appeals to my own desire to exhaust the physical body. I know not all teachers of this style will be the same but unfortunately the one I met was the man who did that weird dragging me to the end of my mat adjustment when I was in Boat Pose, which, coupled with his putting on an Indian accent, put me off exploring this method further (see page 140).

22. Yoga Bites and Snacks (as seen on social media)

Not strictly a type of class but mini practice tips and exercises to perhaps strengthen your shoulders or open the hips to prepare for other poses. This is where teachers post snippets of things you can practise, like drills at the gym. I see them as the yoga equivalent of a soundbite. I've never found the time to do anything extra on top of my usual practice, and I don't know many others who have. If it's not built into our actual practice, I just won't do it. These snacks must help some people though because I've seen teachers post them a lot, which I'm guessing means there's a demand for them.

23. Yoga Nidra

I'm a huge fan of Nidra. It's the best thing ever and everyone should try it. It's a powerful relaxation technique that takes about twenty minutes to do but you can do it for longer. Yoga Nidra means 'yoga sleep' but, rather than falling asleep, it's designed to make us feel like we've 'fallen awake' and feel utterly rested in body but completely alert in the mind – a bit like the feeling after a power nap. The only way to fully understand how this feels is to try it. There are MP3 downloads and YouTube tutorials online. You obviously have to enjoy listening to the voice of the person leading or it can destroy the experience. I recommend those by Uma Dinsmore-Tuli whose workshops I have attended in real life. I love her use of language and her voice. It's her way of leading this practice that inspires the way I teach Nidra and everyone always loves it. They can be found at: yoganidranetwork.org.

Additional Resources and Where to Get Help

Yoga

Yoga Teachers' Union
A branch of the Independent Workers' Union of Great Britain.
https://yogateachersunion.co.uk/

SOAS Centre of Yoga Studies
Department dedicated to Yoga Studies at SOAS, University of London.
https://www.soas.ac.uk/yoga-studies/

The Minded Institute
Training body providing yoga therapy education to yoga and health professionals to work with mental and physical health conditions.
https://themindedinstitute.com/

The Yogic Studies Podcast
Conversations and interviews with yoga scholars and practitioners. https://podcast.yogicstudies.com/

The Yoga is Dead Podcast
A podcast that explores power, privilege, fair pay, harassment, race, cultural appropriation and capitalism in the yoga and wellness worlds.
https://www.yogaisdeadpodcast.com/home

The OMPowerment Project
A charity that offers refugees free training in yoga, community-centred healing and tools for trauma so that they can support their own communities.
https://ompower.org/

Recovery

Mental health charities

Mind
https://www.mind.org.uk/

Rethink Mental Illness
https://www.rethink.org/

Young Minds
https://www.youngminds.org.uk/

The Samaritans
24-hour helpline for mental health support.
https://www.samaritans.org/

Eating disorder and addiction charities

Beat Eating Disorders
https://www.beateatingdisorders.org.uk/

Anorexia and Bulimia Care
https://www.anorexiabulimiacare.org.uk/

Overeaters Anonymous
12-step fellowship for those struggling with any form of disordered eating.
https://www.oagb.org.uk/

Alcoholics Anonymous
12-Step fellowship for anyone who has a desire to stop drinking.
https://www.alcoholics-anonymous.org.uk/

Domestic Violence

Refuge
https://www.refuge.org.uk/

Women's Aid
https://www.womensaid.org.uk/

Victim Support
Charity that supports victims to report a crime confidentially.
https://www.victimsupport.org.uk

LGBTQ+

Lesbian and Gay Switchboard
https://switchboard.lgbt/

Galop
LGBT anti-abuse charity.
https://galop.org.uk/

The Outside Project
LGBT refuge in London.
https://lgbtiqoutside.org/

LGBT Foundation
https://lgbt.foundation/

Stonewall
National campaigning and lobbying organization.
https://www.stonewall.org.uk/

UK Black Pride
Europe's largest celebration for African, Asian, Middle Eastern, Latin American and Caribbean-heritage LGBTQI+ people.
https://www.ukblackpride.org.uk/

Sarbat
LGBT Sikh organization.
https://www.sarbat.net/

House of Rainbow
Support for people of faith.
https://www.houseofrainbow.org/

Imaan
LGBT Muslim organization.
https://imaanlondon.wordpress.com/

Support for people of colour

Ashna
Intersectional counseling, psychotherapy, consultancy and training.
https://www.aashna.uk/

Sistah Space
Community-based domestic abuse services for African heritage women and girls.
https://www.sistahspace.org/

Nafsiyat Intercultural Therapy Centre
Charity offering therapy in over 20 languages.
https://www.nafsiyat.org.uk/

The Black African and Asian Therapy Network
https://www.baatn.org.uk/

Naz
Sexual health.
https://www.naz.org.uk/

Endnotes

1   https://www.mind.org.uk/information-support/types-of-mental-health-problems/eating-problems/types-of-eating-disorders/#Anorexia

2   https://www.beateatingdisorders.org.uk/media-centre/eating-disorder-statistics/

3   Bessell Van Der Kolk, *The Body Keeps the Score: Mind, Brain and Body in the Transformation of Trauma*, Penguin, 2015

4   Gabor Maté, *In the Realm of Hungry Ghosts: Close Encounters with Addiction*, Vermilion, 2018

5   Melanie Cooper, *Teaching Yoga, Adjusting Asana: A handbook for students and teachers*, YogaWords, 2013

6   Eddie Stern, *One Simple Thing: A New Look at the Science of Yoga and How It Can Transform Your Life*, North Point Press, 2019

7   Edwin Bryant, *Yoga Sutras of Patañjali*, North Point Press, 2009

8   B.K.S. Iyengar, *Light on Yoga*, Schocken Books, 1996

9   https://www.bbc.co.uk/news/world-asia-28755509

10   ibid.

11   ibid.

12   https://thewire.in/politics/sanskrit-heritage-politics-government

13   Richard Freeman, *The Mirror of Yoga: Awakening the Intelligence of Body and Mind*, Shambhala Publications Inc, 2012

14   www.newyorker.com/news/news-desk/yoga-reconsiders-the-role-of-the-guru-in-the-age-of-metoo

15   ibid.

16 www.yogajournal.com/lifestyle/sexual-assault-in-the-ashtanga-yoga-community/

17 matthewremski.com/wordpress/sharaths-statement-on-pattabhi-joiss-assaults-context-links-notes/

18 https://thewalrus.ca/yogas-culture-of-sexual-abuse-nine-women-tell-their-stories/

19 Matthew Remski, *Practice And All Is Coming: Abuse, Cult Dynamics, And Healing In Yoga And Beyond*, Embodied Wisdom Publishing, 2019

20 matthewremski.com/wordpress/sharaths-statement-on-pattabhi-joiss-assaults-context-links-notes/

21 www.kinoyoga.com/why-ashtanga-yoga-still-matters-at-least-to-me-by-kino-macgregor/

22 matthewremski.com/wordpress/sharaths-statement-on-pattabhi-joiss-assaults-context-links-notes/

23 www.newyorker.com/news/news-desk/yoga-reconsiders-the-role-of-the-guru-in-the-age-of-metoo

24 Joan Didion, *The Year of Magical Thinking*, Knopf Publishing Group, 2005

25 Norman Blair, *Brightening Our Inner Skies: Yin and Yoga*, MicMac Margins, 2016

26 www.huffingtonpost.co.uk/entry/yoga-whiteness_uk_5e2b2f-07c5b67d8874b146fa

27 Renni Eddo-Lodge, *Why I'm No Longer Talking to White People About Race*, Bloomsbury Publishing, 2018

28 https://nadiagilani.co.uk/journal/engaged-yoga

29 Thích Nhất Hạnh *How to Relax*, Rider, 2016

30 www.beateatingdisorders.org.uk/about-beat/policy-work/policy-and-best-practice-reports/prevalence-in-the-uk/

31 Kehinde Andrews, *Back to Black: Retelling Black Radicalism for the 21st Century*, Zed Books, 2018

32 https://podcasts.apple.com/be/podcast/136-revolution-is-possible-with-prof-kehinde-andrews/id1212064750?i=1000476970164

33 https://bmjopen.bmj.com/content/10/1/e031848

34 www.adam-buxton.co.uk/podcasts/36

35 www.youtube.com/watch?v=MB5NqfLgpdQ

36 https://yogateachersunion.co.uk/
37 www.yogawithnorman.co.uk/space/c16a5320fa475530d-
    9583c34fd356ef5/pdfs/lets_talk_about._._._.pdf
38 www.yogawithnorman.co.uk/space/c16a5320fa475530d9583c34fd
    356ef5/pdfs/Things_Can_Be_Done_Differently_final_september.pdf
39 www.hols.org.uk/
40 https://butiyoga.com/blogs/news/the-buti-truth
41 www.5rhythms.com/
42 https://thepoweryogaco.com/about/
43 https://moveyourframe.com/classes/power-yoga/

Acknowledgements

Lady Gaga once described songwriting as being like open-heart surgery. I relate. When you're writing from deep inside of you, it can feel like having your heart ripped out of your chest. It happened to me. Writing this book broke me down at times but it also gave me life. And just as that first yoga class in 1996 changed me, so too has the process of writing this book.

Behind every author there is an army of heroes who help get the book done. Here's mine: Firstly, thank you to my agent Abi Fellows for finding me, taking care of me and turning my world upside down in the best possible way. Your passion, enthusiasm and unwavering belief in this project carried me through.

Thank you to Carole Tonkinson for your vision and taking a chance on me. Thank you Martha Burley for your sensitivity, attention to detail and all-round brilliance every step of the way. Thank you Tiana-Jane Dunlop for bowling me over with your design skills and making me a cover star. Thanks also to everyone at Bluebird for your creativity, ideas and shouting from the rooftops on my behalf.

Thank you to Norman Blair, Amani Eke and Gingi Lee for

being generous with your time. Thanks also to Amanda Graziano, Lauren Munday and Lucy Penrose for sharing your stories.

Thank you Rachel Anderson, Ross Benzie, Cis O'Boyle, Samantha Chambers, Sarah Cretch and John Park for friendship. Thank you to Stella Duffy for always saying the right thing.

Special thanks to Kevin Braddock and Emma Warren for companionship, encouragement, sunset gazing and soirées on the Magic Bench. Thank you also to Janos Verebes-Weisz for listening and giving me things to think about. I couldn't have done it without you.

Thank you to anyone who has come to practise with me online, at festivals, in offices, yoga studios, hair salons, leisure centres, in parks, city farms and back rooms in community centres. And special thanks to students I've written about anonymously. If you see yourself, your story needed telling.

Big thanks to my family, especially Farrakh Gilani, for always looking out for me and Haider Gilani, for teaching me what unconditional love is.

Dear reader of this book, thank you for giving this a go. Writing this book was like wrestling with a monster of words spilling out of me, growing bigger than I could contain at times. The biggest lesson I learnt was that if I gave myself to the story, the story would give itself to me until I was ready to give it away. It belongs to you now.

In the end, Tasneem Gilani to whom I owe most things. Thank you for reminding me who I am, for always having my back and being there when I need to come home. I love you Ammi Ji.

About the Author

Nadia Gilani is a writer and yoga teacher. She worked as a news journalist for a decade before teaching yoga and meditation. With extensive experience of working with people from all walks of life, Nadia is deeply committed to making yoga as inclusive as possible. Her approach to teaching is contemporary while maintaining a deep respect for the ancient practice.

@theyogadissident

About the author